rooted
THE DOWN TO EARTH BASICS OF WELLNESS

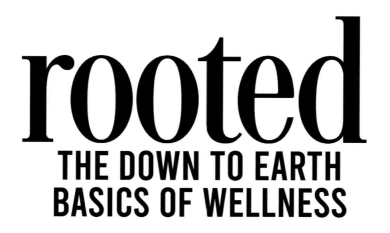

rooted
THE DOWN TO EARTH BASICS OF WELLNESS

AMANDA BRINK HULL

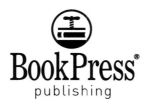

Copyright © 2025 by Amanda Brink Hull. All rights reserved.

No portion of this book may be reproduced, stored in a retrieval system, or transmitted in any form or by any means—electronic, mechanical, photocopy, recording, scanning, or other—except for brief quotations in critical reviews or articles, without prior written permission of the publisher. Requests to the publisher for permission or information should be submitted via email at info@bookpresspublishing.com.

Any requests or questions for the editor should be submitted to him directly at hullhealth22@gmail.com.

Published in Des Moines, Iowa, by:

Bookpress Publishing
P.O. Box 71532
Des Moines, IA 50325
www.BookpressPublishing.com

Publisher's Cataloging-in-Publication Data

Names: Hull, Amanda Brink, author.
Title: Rooted : the down-to-earth basics of wellness / Amanda Brink Hull.
Description: Includes bibliographical references. | Des Moines, IA: Bookpress Publishing, 2025.
Identifiers: LCCN: 2025905382 | ISBN: 978-1-960259-35-6
Subjects: LCSH Health--Popular works. | Self-care, Health--Popular works. | Nutrition--Popular works. | Cooking. | Self-help. | BISAC SELF-HELP / Personal Growth / Success | HEALTH & FITNESS / Diet & Nutrition / General | COOKING / Health & Healing / General
Classification: LCC RA776.95 .H85 2025 | DDC 613--dc23

First Edition
Printed in the United States of America
10 9 8 7 6 5 4 3 2 1

CONTENTS

1   Cultivating Rich Beginnings 1

2   Rooted in Small-Town Iowa 9

3   Active Living: Embracing Exercise and Functional Movements 14

4   Chores to Cheer: Finding Joy in Work and Play 25

5   Nourishing Wellness: The Power of Food and Nutrition 32

6   Zen in Motion: Stress Management Techniques 75

7   Recharge and Renew: Rest and Relaxation Strategies 92

8   Conquering Healthy Challenges: Personal Growth and Thriving 98

9   Dollars and Sense: Financial Fitness 108

10   Harmonious Living: Striking a Balance among Work,
Home, and Life Demands 123

11   Connections Count: Cultivating Relationships and
Social Interaction 141

12   Unveiling Authenticity: The Art of Being You 156

13   Forever Curious: The Journey of Always Learning 167

14   Mindful Navigation: Being Aware in Your Environment 179

15   Guidance in Wellness: Navigating Medical Advice with Confidence 201

16   Lasting Impressions: In the End 225

17   Final Thoughts: Walking the Walk and Living Wellness 234

      Notes 238

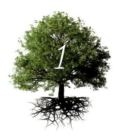

Cultivating Rich Beginnings

I was just shy of being a teenager and the oldest of four sisters—myself, Sara, Katie, and Andrea—all spaced evenly three years apart in age. We all sat at our large, rectangular kitchen table, except for the youngest, "Andie," who was eating chunks of banana in the old wooden highchair that we were all blessed to have used through the years. Our mom hovered over the stove, tending to the large, silver pressure cooker that sat steaming on one of the gas burners. None of us were smiling. We all knew who was about to come through the kitchen door.

Our father was a strong man. He was about three inches shy of six feet but had a stocky frame fit from being an active outdoorsman and his laborious job at the local cooperative. While most men would have used a forklift, my father preferred to load bags of grain onto trucks by hand, sometimes one on each shoulder, just for the workout. He was a hard worker, and it showed. He was also a quiet man, but his dark hair, piercing blue eyes, and smile would immediately put you at ease. I've often wondered if his lack of words and the large amount of time he spent outdoors was the result of living in a small house surrounded by five females.

From the kitchen table, we would frequently watch him work in the larger of two pristine gardens through the old farmhouse window. His loose work jeans were always held up with the leather belt that proudly displayed his nickname "Barney" on the back. Most of the t-shirts he wore were old and stained, which our mom would often criticize by asking him to change into one of his cleaner shirts whenever we were expecting company or going out in public. In the summer months, his stained t-shirts would show the signs of a good sweat while he worked outdoors on those hot and humid Iowa days. The heat never seemed to bother him.

As we reluctantly sat around the kitchen table that day, we could see Dad approaching the window, walking from the south garden. The sound of his footsteps in sloppy old workbooks was in rhythm with the clicking handles of the two five-gallon buckets he was carrying. His voice penetrated the window screen as he walked by, "Suzie, I am coming in!" This was our warning that in a matter of seconds, he would be stepping through the kitchen door to deliver the contents of those big buckets.

Dad appeared in the kitchen doorway and, without hesitation, headed straight to the kitchen table, turned both buckets upside down to empty what was inside into one large pile in front of us, and proudly exclaimed, "Get to shucking, girls."

And there we sat in front of a heaping mound of fresh garden peas, all ten gallons of them. Andrea was too little to help. So that left me, Sara, and Katie to do all the work. Every year, it seemed like an impossible task as we stared at the mountain of bright green pea pods in front of us. We absolutely hated shucking peas. But, despite our reluctance, each of us took one pea pod, split it open with our thumbs, and pushed the ripe round peas out into recycled plastic ice cream buckets, discarding the pod in a separate pile that we would later take out to either the chickens or pigs. Shucking peas was absolute torture. Our thumbs would always be sore and stained green after this annual family affair.

I remember trying to bargain with Dad once, offering to use my own money to buy the family frozen peas from the grocery store to avoid the whole pea harvesting process altogether. Buying frozen peas seemed well worth the investment if it meant not having to shuck peas ever again.

Sometimes, Dad would head back out to the garden to tend to the sweet corn, check on the potato crop, or pull weeds. And other times, he would join us at the table to help speed up the pea-shucking process so Mom could get on with canning and freezing.

Mom was still standing at the stove supervising our work while she pulled out the steaming glass jars of green beans from the pressure cooker with a metal tong. Once all the jars of green beans were organized on the wooden butcher block that sat just left of the stove, she inspected the jars one by one to make sure that each lid was properly sealed for storage. Earlier that same morning, the three of us older girls and Mom washed and cut two full buckets of green beans, which were now being canned so we could enjoy them in the coming fall and winter months.

This is how the Brink family spent our summers. And Dad loved every single minute. From tilling and planting in the spring to weeding all summer long and then harvesting in late summer into early fall. Dad absolutely adored his two gardens, which seemed like they took up one-third of our three-acre homestead. Mom always complained that two gardens were way too much; one would be plenty. But Dad insisted on planting two each year, and he always got his way.

Every summer, without fail, our neighbors and close acquaintances received the surplus of fruits and vegetables from Dad's gardens. They were always very thankful, and Dad took great pride in gifting some of the most beautiful produce ever grown. Year after year, there was an abundance beyond what the six of us could ever eat ourselves. Our family was rich in fruits and vegetables, and the overabundance was a direct result of the discipline and hard work both Mom and Dad instilled in the four of us girls. This was how we "food prepped" back in the 1980s on our little acreage that sat on a gravel road just outside of a very tiny Iowa town.

Dad was not a farmer, though the acreage in which we lived was surrounded by fields of corn and soybeans. Mom and Dad did not own any farmland, like most of our neighbors. But just because Dad

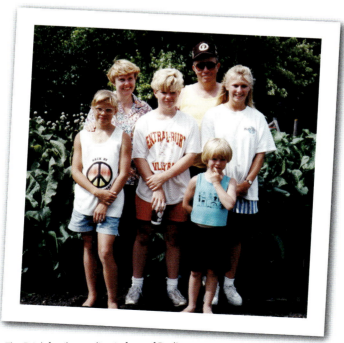

The Brink family standing in front of Dad's horseradish patch in the garden.

was not a traditional farmer, did not mean he did not work like one. His job at the Fenton Co-Op gave him the opportunity to work for a lot of local farmers, hauling grain, delivering feed, and spraying northern Iowa farm fields in the cooperative's TerraGator. He looked like a farmer and probably worked harder than any farmer we knew.

Dad could carry two five-gallon buckets of water from the house (which is where the water hose was) to the outbuildings just as easily as he could carry the two buckets full of fresh garden peas. When one of us girls was asked to take water down to the chickens, it was a struggle just to carry half of a bucket of water one hundred yards to the white miniature barn we called the chicken house. But we did it, one-half bucket at a time. Eventually, we got stronger as we got older and could muster the five-gallon pails with a few stops to rest, giving our muscles and grip strength a much-needed break.

Not only did Dad have two bountiful gardens to care for, but he also had a passion for hunting and was good at it. His expertise extended across various game, from pheasants to wild turkeys and white-tailed deer. Proficient with shotguns, rifles, muzzleloaders, and compound bows, he displayed remarkable skill in his pursuits. Over the years, I bet Dad walked a million miles through fields and timber. He treasured being outdoors, pursuing wild game, and the patience and expertise it took to have a successful hunt—and we ate every bite of prey that he brought home. Slow-cooked deer roasts with canned green beans and baked potatoes dug up from the garden were a family favorite after church on Sundays. I would go back to those days in a heartbeat.

Our summers growing up on those three acres were filled with potato planting, weed pulling, corn shucking, pea picking, jelly making, dirt hoeing, chicken butchering, and brush cleaning fun. It was our way of life, and we didn't think twice about it. Mom and Dad told us it built character and a solid work ethic.

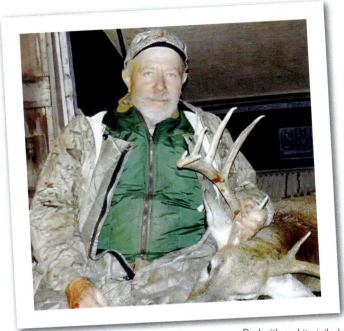

Dad with a white-tailed buck after a succesful hunt.

Some chores were easier than others and some seemed like downright abuse. But no matter how easy or how hard, we made the most of it, and sometimes we even had fun (though we hated to admit it) while we worked. The conversations we sisters would find ourselves having would either lead to laughs or arguments. Both of which would distract us from the task at hand. There were times that our joint work turned into an all-out sibling rivalry because one sister wasn't pulling her weight, which usually resulted in one of us tattling to Mom that the job was not being done correctly by another.

Physical work was a big part of growing up, and you were never too young to be assigned responsibilities. Not only did we have work to do in the garden and during harvest season, but there were plenty of other things to do in the house and outside around the acreage.

When the weather was nice enough, we hung wet clothes out on the clothesline to dry and helped Mom fold laundry. And, when Dad needed help digging post holes for fencing, we were right there beside him to scoop the loose dirt from the deep holes made by the manual post hole digger that he would strongly turn into the ground. All four of us girls did our fair share of shoveling chicken and goat manure too, and all year round we helped in the house by dusting and vacuuming. There was always work to do, and Mom and Dad made sure we kept busy.

Back in the pea-picking days, we did not have the luxury of a dishwasher, so dishes needed to be washed by hand. This fell on us girls to do each night, even if it meant using a stepstool to reach the faucet because we weren't quite tall enough. When Sara and I were the only ones old enough to do dishes, we rotated every night, one night on, one night off. But then, when Katie grew into the post-dinner ritual by getting to a height where she was tall enough to reach the faucet from the step stool, the three of us voted on a weekly dishwashing schedule. That meant one full week of scrubbing pots and pans, washing plates, and hand-drying drinking glasses. But it also meant two full weeks off, leaving us able to help Mom and Dad with other chores, do homework, or have the freedom to play.

We prayed for a riding lawn mower just like we prayed for a dishwasher, but back in those days, Mom and Dad could not afford either, so we push-mowed the lawn, which was a lot of work considering that Dad's gardens and the small grove just north of the house left a lot of thick green grass for us to mow. Sometimes, mowing the lawn took two days as we divided the job into sections, taking turns with the push mower. But when the job was done, the yard looked amazing, and the smell of fresh-cut grass inspired all of us to stay outside and soak in our hard work. Sometimes, we would simply relax in the front yard by sitting on an old porch swing that was set up underneath a big shady tree, which also accommodated a tire swing Dad hung up for us. Other times, we celebrated the newly cut grass with the whole family (all six of us) playing a casual game of softball.

It didn't matter how it all got done or if each task ended in smiles or frustration; the outcome was always well worth it. We all appreciated our beautiful homestead and the amazing home-cooked meals that our family shared around the same table where we shucked mountains of peas and cut heaping hills of green beans. We were incredibly fortunate to enjoy such great food every single day of the year. And we were even more fortunate to have each other's company.

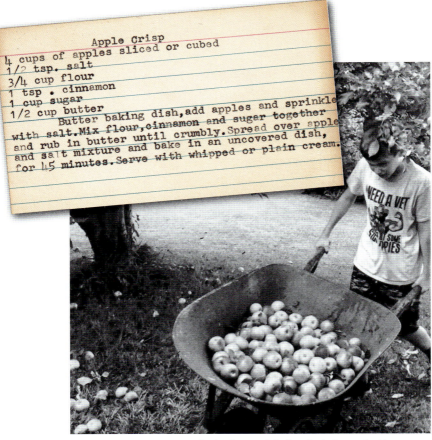

```
                Apple Crisp
4 cups of apples sliced or cubed
1/2 tsp. salt
3/4 cup flour
1 tsp . cinnamon
1 cup sugar
1/2 cup butter
    Butter baking dish, add apples and sprinkle
with salt. Mix flour, cinnamon and sugar together
and rub in butter until crumbly. Spread over apple
and salt mixture and bake in an uncovered dish,
for 45 minutes. Serve with whipped or plain cream.
```

A wheelbarrow full of apples being pushed by our son, Cameron, that were picked from one of Mom & Dad's trees.

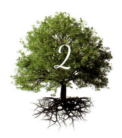

Rooted in Small-Town Iowa

Fenton, Iowa (population 300) sits just 6 miles northeast of the acreage where we were raised. From our house, you had to travel on two to three miles of gravel roads to get into town, depending on what route you chose. Our vehicles were never clean, always full of dust, mud, or frozen slush, contingent on the season. Once you reached the blacktop on the southern edge of town, you'd come across Maple Street, which is the "main street" that runs north and south straight through the middle of town. Maple Street is only seven blocks long with the grain elevator at the very north end. This is where Dad worked. To get to the Fenton Co-Op, you'd drive through town, past the Methodist church, library, post office, bank, and the legendary NorthStar Restaurant and Lounge. Fenton also had a funeral home and a Lutheran church, but they were located off the main drag and on one of Fenton's side streets.

The Fenton gas station (nicknamed "The Pop Shop") was on the northeast corner of town and offered soft-serve ice cream. Oftentimes, Dad would drive into Fenton just to get a quart of this special treat for us to share, along with one small package of whole cashews that he would gently crush up using a hammer once at home. The broken cashew pieces would be used as a topping along with the chocolate syrup in a can found in the back of our refrigerator.

Fenton had one place to buy clothing: the Mercantile. It was a consignment shop where Mom liked to visit often, buying our clothes for school. Rarely did we get anything new. Across from the Mercantile was the grocery store, which was a typical small-town deli-style store offering bare necessities. It was also where we kids would walk three hot blocks from the swimming pool in the summer months to buy cheap candy. The Fenton Community Swimming Pool, which does not exist anymore, was on the west edge of town and overlooked cornfields to the west and the grain elevator to the north. Today, the town is simply too small to support any retail business, and so the gas station, Mercantile, and little grocery store are all abandoned and empty.

Fenton, Iowa, was one of three towns that consolidated to form the Sentral Community School District. Yes, Sentral spelled with an "S." The towns of Lone Rock and Burt were straight west of Fenton and joined forces that made up the school district. Before the consolidation, the school was known as Sentral of Fenton. The school mascot was the Satellite, which is almost as odd as spelling Sentral with an "S." Our school colors were red and white, and we were amusingly known in our district as the Sentral Satellites. You can find the large red and white mascot hanging in the NorthStar today. After the three towns combined into one district, Sentral changed its mascot to a Spartan sporting red and gold colors. We were then the Sentral-Burt Spartans starting my 7th grade year.

The school building itself sat in the middle of a field between

ROOTED IN SMALL-TOWN IOWA

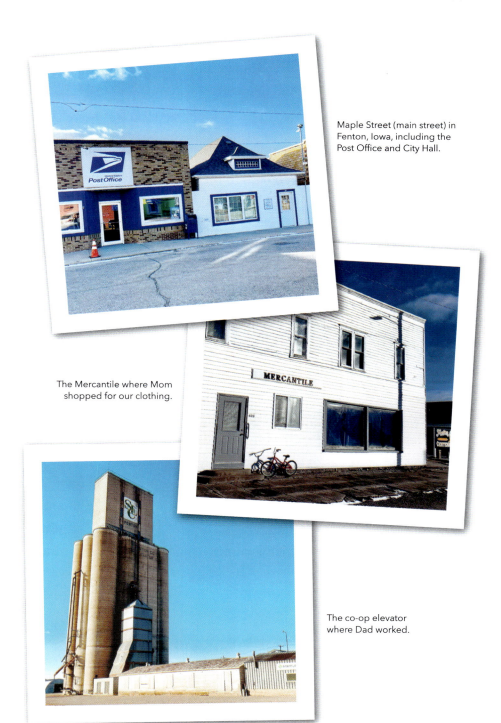

Maple Street (main street) in Fenton, Iowa, including the Post Office and City Hall.

The Mercantile where Mom shopped for our clothing.

The co-op elevator where Dad worked.

Fenton and Lone Rock and accommodated all students from kindergarten through twelfth grade. Because all grades K-12 were in one building, there was a period of a few years when all four of us sisters attended school in the single-level red brick building at the same time. Class sizes at Sentral ranged between twenty and thirty kids. I had twenty-seven kids in my graduating class of 1993.

There were just over one hundred students in the whole high school, which consumed the south end of the building along with the art room, gymnasium, music rooms, and cafeteria. The elementary school was located on the north end of the building, with one classroom for each grade; kindergarten was at the very end of the hallway. Junior high students had lockers in-between the elementary hall and where the high school lockers were located and shared classrooms with the high school students, which were not broken out by grade but by subject. The playground and baseball field sat east of the building, and the grass football field to the west. It was a condensed campus, simple, streamlined, and very country.

Due to the small size of our school, students had the opportunity to actively participate in a wide range of activities, whether they were interested in athletics or academic groups. I took full advantage of this and was part of the volleyball and track teams, cheered on the basketball cheerleading squad, played the clarinet and bass clarinet in concert band, sang in choir, served on the annual staff, was vice president of the graduating class of 1993, and was nominated president of the student council my senior year. Sentral was so small that the football coach even asked me if I wanted to join the football team due to my athletic strength and can-do attitude; and he was serious! The Spartan football team eventually transitioned to an eight-member team a few years after I graduated because the school just didn't have the numbers for a competitive eleven-member team. Eight-member football is common today for many small-town school districts.

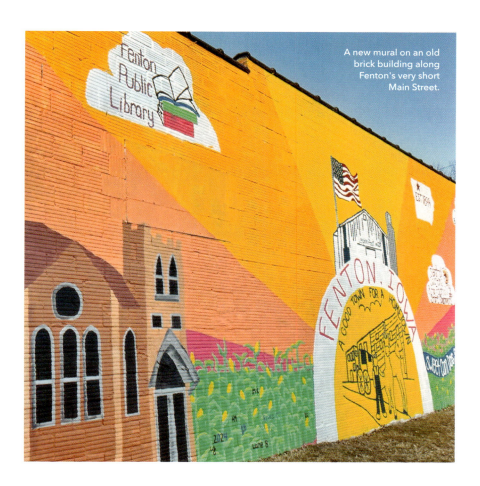

A new mural on an old brick building along Fenton's very short Main Street.

I loved my childhood, from being a young girl shucking peas at the kitchen table with my sisters to the experiences I was blessed to have in a small high school. Life was simple back then in Fenton, Iowa. People were truly connected in meaningful ways—not by social media—because the technology did not exist back then. Families ate dinner together at night and talked about their day. Playing outside was a normal part of our lives for both children and adults. Sunday school and church were what you did every Sunday morning. Everyone worked hard because we had to, and that is what made life back then all so rewarding.

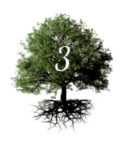

Active Living:
Embracing Exercise and Functional Movement

Growing up, we had to physically move to get things done. Exercise was naturally part of our lives. No one really scheduled time to "exercise" because our days were full of physical tasks that gave us a good sweat, enhanced our endurance, and developed farm-strong muscles. Accomplishing a good list of chores each day also made us sleep better at night too. Chores were functional fitness and a healthy part of daily living.

All the chores we did growing up made us good athletes in high school, disciplined in hard work, more confident to try new tasks, and increased how adventurous we were in play. Chores also helped build a healthy foundation for all four of us girls as we became adults with families of our own, not afraid of putting in a conscious effort to get things done and making sure our children all knew and appreciated the value of a solid work ethic.

Today, society has become much more sedentary than the days

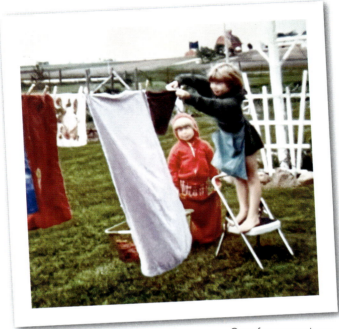

One of our many chores... hanging clothes out on the line with my sister.

of my childhood. Advancements in technology and in the food industry have given us conveniences and countless reasons to be inactive, relying on others to do the work for us. Did you know that the average person sits an average of 6.5 to 8 hours every day? We sit at desks all day at office jobs and then come home and sit more in front of a television or on our digital devices. We walk and bike far less and drive more to wherever we need to go. Kids take the bus versus walking to and from school, even if it is only a few blocks away. Online shopping makes it way too convenient to have items delivered to our front doorsteps (while we sit on our sofas) and allows us to avoid physical outings to the store. Food delivery services provide us with a double whammy by replacing home-cooked meals with less nutritious choices like fast food and fried foods and keep us from working in our kitchens creating healthier options. Plus, food delivery services can be more expensive than making our own food, which taps into our financial well-being.

Convenience is habit forming. Conveniences have become much too common and have created an addiction and very strong dependency on instant gratification. The opportunity for convenience makes it too easy to use "time" as an excuse. When time is an excuse, the first two things we cut out of our busy schedules are exercise (aka movement) and making our own food, which are two of the most important elements humans need to live our best lives. Time has become a very common excuse; however, keep in mind the "time" we spend on technology, endlessly surfing the web or unconsciously scrolling through social media. The trade-off in how we spend our time is evident in the current rates of obesity and the prevalence of chronic illnesses. We all have time for what is important if we make time. How we spend our time is a choice; it is simply a matter of how we prioritize our time. Time is not an excuse.

Sedentary lifestyles pose some serious risks to both our physical and mental health. Here are only seven for you to consider:

1. *OBESITY:* Lack of physical activity leads to weight gain. While body positivity is important and seems to be a popular movement these days, it's also important to acknowledge that being overweight comes with challenges and discomforts. Being overweight or obese limits our abilities in so many ways. Plus, it increases the risk of heart disease, diabetes, and certain cancers.

2. *CARDIOVASCULAR PROBLEMS:* Heart disease is the leading cause of death in the United States, with over 700,000 deaths per year, most of which are preventable. Sedentary behavior contributes to high blood pressure, elevated cholesterol levels, and an increased risk of heart attack and stroke.

3. *MUSCLE AND JOINT PROBLEMS:* Muscle is valuable real estate, and we need to protect it. Use it or lose it. And so, a sedentary lifestyle leads to muscle weakness, stiffness, and decreased flexibility. It can also contribute to joint pain and increase the risk of conditions such as osteoporosis and arthritis.

4. *DECREASED MOBILITY:* Being inactive leads to a decline in overall mobility and functional abilities, making everyday tasks more challenging and increasing the risk of falls and injuries. The ability to bend down to tie your shoes or pick up items from the ground illustrates how mobility gives us independence (especially as we grow older).

5. *MENTAL HEALTH ISSUES:* Sedentary behavior has been linked to an increased risk of depression, anxiety, and cognitive decline.

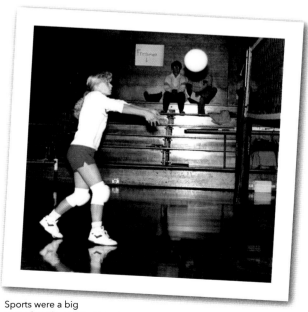

Sports were a big part of our lives growing up.

Whenever one of us girls was having a bad day, Mom would tell us to go outside and take a walk (which, to this day, she still does faithfully every day, rain or shine). Physical activity is important for promoting mental well-being and reducing stress.

6. *POOR POSTURE:* Spending extended periods of time sitting or lying down can contribute to poor posture, which causes back and neck pain. And, lack of activity reduces muscle mass, which plays an important role in maintaining posture. Poor posture can contribute to an aged appearance. With good posture, we can look years younger!

7. *REDUCED LIFESPAN:* Regular physical activity is linked to longevity and a lower risk of premature death. Studies have shown that a sedentary lifestyle is associated with a shorter lifespan, and who wants that?

Every single one of the effects listed above (and more) of living a sedentary lifestyle is preventable, and none of them sound like a fun way to live.

Humans are built to stand upright, and our bodies are designed to move—not to sit at a desk or in front of a screen for eight hours a day, as many of us do in today's modern world. That's why it's incredibly important for us to incorporate movement and exercise into our daily routines. Maintaining an active lifestyle is crucial to preserve both physical and mental health along with reducing the risks associated with sedentary behavior. Simply put, without movement, our bodies become weak and dysfunctional.

I always like to compare our bodies to a river. Rivers are the lifeblood of their surroundings, always in motion, bringing vitality wherever they flow. Life is found in and around rivers. When a body of water becomes sedentary, water molecules become stagnant, and the oxygen is depleted. Your circulatory, respiratory, lymphatic, and digestive systems all require movement to operate optimally. Optimal health flourishes when movement becomes a regular part of our daily rhythm. So, move more and get all your body's systems flowing like a vibrant river—filling them (and yourself) with life!

When my sisters and I were little, we constantly used our imaginations along with our physical abilities. Many times, our inspiration came from characters we would see in the movies or on TV. I remember pretending to be Cinderella, the poor servant girl, down on my hands and knees, scrubbing the rough cement block outside our back door with an old rag. No one asked me to do it; I put myself to work and had fun scrubbing away, imagining I was the beautiful princess. By the time I finished, the eight-by-ten slab of concrete had transformed from murky dark gray to a clean, white-washed finish. I used various rags from the rag drawer in our bathroom, an old scrub brush, and a bucket of soapy water—just like Cinderella in the Disney movie while her stepsisters were out having fun. I was no Cinderella, and my sisters were not at all like the stepsisters in the movie, but what an imagination!

There were also times when we girls would all put on dance leotards (sometimes with tights and leg warmers) and pretend we were in the circus. We loved watching the annual *Ringling Brothers Barnum & Bailey Circus* on TV. It motivated us to get out and perform (to the best of our ability) gymnastics. We would do somersaults, cartwheels, and attempt front flips in the yard. Sometimes, our blond-colored horse, Candy, would even make it into a circus routine or two as one of us would attempt to stand up on her back and balance while another sister would lead her around the yard. Mom and Dad watched with affectionate adoration as we performed every daring trick.

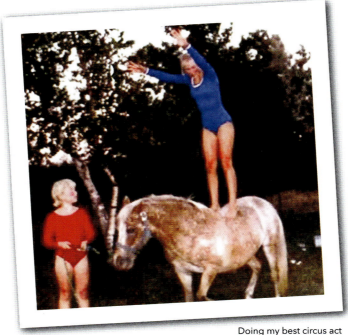

Doing my best circus act while standing on our horse Candy.

My leotard was not just limited to circus play. I also wore it to imitate She-Ra from *Masters of the Universe: He-Man and She-Ra*. These two muscle-bound cartoon heroes protected the universe from the power of Grayskull. She-Ra was strong and beautiful, and I wanted to be just like her (probably more so than Cinderella), saving victims from all sorts of peculiar circumstances. So, sporting my leotard, I would ride my yellow bike with the banana seat up and down the gravel roads, scouting for humans in trouble. I never found any. I even named my big, long-haired yellow and white domesticated cat "Cringer." Cringer was He-Man's trusty side-kick cat in the cartoon series.

Looking back to my childhood and our daily routines on that acreage outside of Fenton, Iowa, we came to appreciate the significant value of staying physically active. We gained a genuine understanding of the advantages of exercise, even though we didn't label our chores and playing outdoors as exercise back then. My three younger sisters and I learned that "a body in motion stays in motion," and that the importance of getting outside and engaging in physical activity is critical as we age and can even be fun—really fun. Engaging in hard work helped us appreciate exercise and what our bodies and minds are truly capable of. It also taught us that there is nothing wrong with a little dirt and sweat. It has also taught me that as we get older, muscle is far more beneficial to us than just appearance—it contributes to overall strength and well-being.

There is a powerful saying that I had printed on the back of a hooded sweatshirt, which I have proudly worn for years, "Ask your doctor if getting off your ass is right for you." And so, I challenge you to get off your rump and do something. Start today, start now.

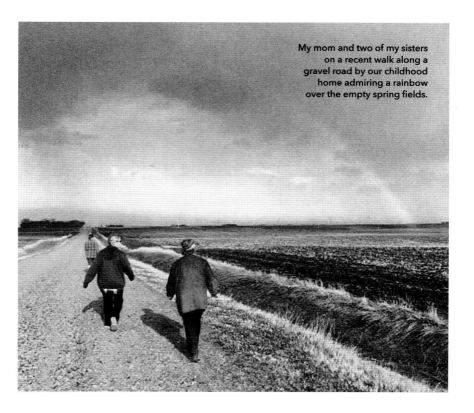

My mom and two of my sisters on a recent walk along a gravel road by our childhood home admiring a rainbow over the empty spring fields.

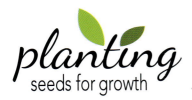 A Harvest of Functional Movements

Before jumping into a new exercise program, check in with your doctor—it's like getting the green light before a big race. And remember, if something hurts, it's your body's way of saying, "Hey, take a breather!" Listen to it and pause.

- **STEP-UPS.** Find a good solid step or bench and get some reps in of simple step-ups. This movement comes in handy if you need a step stool to do dishes or to reach the top shelf in your kitchen cupboard. This movement improves balance and is great for improving lower body strength.

- **FARMER'S CARRY (one bucket or two).** You can also use a dumbbell(s), kettlebell(s), sandbag, or weights of any kind. This movement mimics that of carrying suitcases, grocery bags, a gas can, or water jugs. It is great for grip strength, shoulder, and arm strength and wonderful to improve balance.

- **SLED PUSH & SLED PULLS.** If your gym has a weighted sled, sled pushes and pulls are fantastic for a full-body workout. It's like mowing the lawn with a push mower, tilling the garden, shoveling heavy snow, or pushing a trailer to hitch it to a pickup truck. Even pushing or pulling a wagon full of kids, pets, or groceries can give you a great workout. For a classic touch, wheelbarrows are another excellent way to build strength and endurance!

- **SANDBAG CARRIES.** Like the bags of feed that Dad would throw over his shoulders, get yourself a sandbag and use it to add weight to short walks and incorporate it into workouts. A bag of cat food, dog food, or chicken feed works well too. Sandbags come in many sizes and the weight can be adjusted by the amount of sand you fill it with. You can use it for back squats, front squats, and deadlifts. Sandbag tosses are like shoveling dirt and are great for building core and upper body strength.

• *AIR SQUATS.* No equipment is needed for this movement, which is required for picking peas in the garden or if you need to pick something up off the ground. Squatting is great to build leg muscle strength and being able to squat lowers your chances of injury.

• *PUSH-UPS*. Build arm strength with this simple bodyweight movement that you can even do from your knees. Being able to do push-ups can protect your shoulders and lower back from injuries, and they help with balance and posture. Push-ups are handy if you need to look under your car or get something from underneath a sofa or bed.

• *PUSH-PRESSES.* Grab that sandbag and use both arms to lift it over your head or pick up a dumbbell and use one arm doing alternate shoulder-to-overhead movements with weight. Pushing weight over your head is like putting a bag in the overhead compartment of an airplane or retrieving something from the top shelf of a cupboard.

• *WALKING.* Get outside and just walk. Walking just thirty minutes a day boosts your metabolism and immune system. Walking is a great way to strengthen bones, joints, and muscles. The therapeutic benefits of walking are endless as it relieves stress, improves your mood and cognitive function, aids in better sleep at night, and helps your digestive system run smoothly.

- **BEAR CRAWLS.** Get down on all fours with your butt in the air and walk for a good distance on your hands and feet. This is a wonderful animal-like movement that lengthens your calves and hamstrings and gives your shoulders a good challenge.

- **CRAB WALKS.** Quite the opposite of the bear crawl, the crab walk is a fun way to tighten the glutes and work those abs and arms. Face the sky and use your hands and feet to lift your torso off the ground. Keep your core tight and butt up off the ground. Walk forward or backward and practice balance.

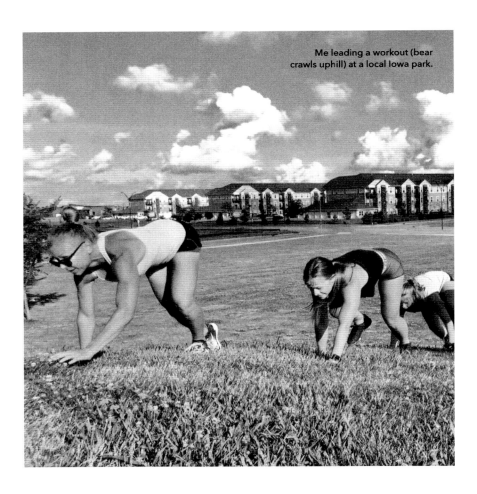

Me leading a workout (bear crawls uphill) at a local Iowa park.

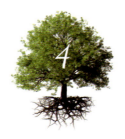

Chores to Cheer:
Finding Joy in Work and Play

    During weekends in the spring, our family would all pack into the car; Mom and Dad in the front seat and all four of us girls in the backseat. Car seats were not a thing, and there were no seatbelt laws back then. Heck, vehicles in the 80s and 90s would not even beep at you to remind you to wear your seatbelt if it wasn't buckled. Sometimes, our Grandma Vuanita would come along too, which would pack seven people in one vehicle. Grandma "Nita" was Mom's mom and was a petite but fiery woman who stood just over five feet tall, with short, auburn hair and bright red lipstick. Since she was kid-sized she could easily either squeeze in the backseat with us by putting Andie on her lap, or she could fit in the front seat with Mom and Dad. Cars back then typically had a bench seat in the front without the console in the middle, so three normal-sized people could easily fit in the front.

    With all of us in one vehicle, we would slowly drive around on the gravel roads near our house for hours, hunting asparagus. All of us attentively peering out the open car windows, trying to spot the signs of asparagus coming up through the tall weeds in the green ditches. We would take empty bread sacks with us and have them ready to fill with fresh wild asparagus. When one of us would spot an old seeded-out asparagus plant, which was the sign there could be baby asparagus spears underneath it or even see the tender baby spears themselves from the road, we would pull the car over to the shoulder, get out, run down into the ditch, and harvest the delicious vegetable that grows wild in Iowa's countryside.

Asparagus hunting was harvesting food to eat, and it was fun. We loved those slow car rides filled with conversation, laughs, and the friendly competition of who could collect the most asparagus in their bread sack. Between all of us, there would be an abundance that we appreciated cooking and eating for dinner that night and usually for many meals afterward. Grandma Nita always got her fair share after the hunt, taking home at least one bread sack full of the nutritious vegetable treat.

Just like we would hunt asparagus, we would also hunt for rocks. Hunting rocks was like hunting for asparagus, driving the same gravel roads at the same slow speeds. But instead of food, we hunted rocks for landscaping purposes. We found our own treasures in field rocks to create borders around flower beds, trees, and for decoration. Sometimes, the rocks we found to bring home were so big they took two people to lift and move. Other times we found pretty rocks that were so small you could fit them in your coat pocket. Mom called these smaller rocks that we would collect "smoothies." She loved smoothies, and often, we would find handfuls of colorful rocks worn smooth (probably over centuries) in her coat pocket. Mom would typically pick up smoothies that caught her eye during her daily walks and later would transfer them to her rock garden on the east end of the house

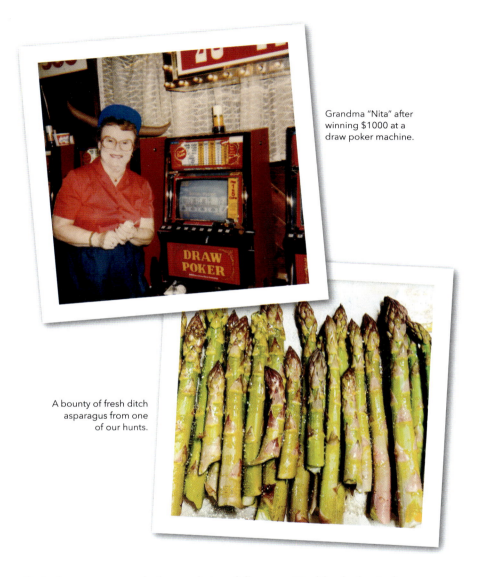

Grandma "Nita" after winning $1000 at a draw poker machine.

A bounty of fresh ditch asparagus from one of our hunts.

that also accompanied a variety of flowers Dad had planted.

Asparagus hunting for food and hunting rocks for landscaping projects were not considered work or even a chore. These were wonderful ways to enjoy the outdoors together, engage in physical activity, and make meaningful use of our time. We viewed these amusing little hobbies as enjoyable rather than laborious tasks, much like Dad saw gardening as a stimulating and rewarding activity.

Discovering happiness in chores benefits both our physical health and mental well-being. Regardless of age, everyone can find activities they are good at and even enjoy. Hunting for asparagus (and rocks) became a cherished family tradition, filled with excitement, much like Dad's passion for gardening and the anticipation of harvesting colorful fruits and vegetables to nourish and share with loved ones.

I encourage you to find creative and fun ways to do household chores. Turn mundane everyday jobs into playful experiences. For instance, when raking leaves, gather them into a huge pile for the whole family to jump in; an amusing way to tidy up the yard. If you're mowing the lawn, challenge yourself to create elaborate patterns like that of a baseball field, then take a moment to admire your work when the job is done. For indoor chores, turn it into a game: assign different tasks to each family member (dusting, vacuuming, folding laundry, doing dishes, etc.), and once all chores are completed using a teamwork approach, reward yourselves with a fun activity. Break out a deck of cards or a board game, enjoy some yummy snacks, and indulge in healthy competition.

Whether you're living solo or with family members, there are ways to find enjoyment in everyday responsibilities. Take cooking, for example; it may feel like a chore to some, but it can also be a source of pleasure and creativity. Instead of viewing it as a work, consider cooking homemade meals as a form of artistic expression. By mentally reframing the chore, you can take pride in the nourishing dishes you create and find great satisfaction in accomplishing something amazing.

For parents, raising children is undoubtedly hard work. Being a parent is a full-time commitment that can feel like a major chore at times. In today's world, it's easy to rely on video games and television as babysitters, but actively engaging with your children is a worthwhile chore and should be a priority (for the sake of your children). These moments are precious and fleeting, and you'll cherish them when your kiddos are all grown up and gone. Spending quality time with your little ones is critical in sharing your wisdom with them and instilling healthy habits that will guide them into adulthood. Engage in conversation, teach them the art of having good discussions and using their manners. Embrace opportunities to shape their future, all while you are creating lasting memories together. Your efforts will not go unnoticed, you will have no regrets, and when your kids are grown, they will thank you for the quality time you spent with them, I promise. Looking back, I deeply cherish those moments with my mom and dad. Now that my kids are grown, I hope they hold the same appreciation for the family time we shared during their childhood and continue to treasure it to this day.

It is astounding that every time we go out to enjoy dinner, there is always a table or two with young children who sit and watch movies or play video games on a cell phone throughout the entire meal, never even looking up to address the waiter or waitress. The parents at the table might briefly interact with their device-dependent children or have light discussions among themselves while eating, unless they, too, are engrossed in their own devices. And, when we are at ballgames or concerts, small toddlers will literally spend hours on an iPad instead of observing what is going on all around them.

Back when I was a kid, I remember Dad taking us to baseball games in Bancroft, Iowa where he grew up and just northeast of Fenton. Grandpa and Grandma Brink still lived in Bancroft at the time, just outside of town. The baseball games Dad took us to were long, and it was hard for us girls to sit still in the stands for an entire nine innings, so we would find a nice grassy area and play catch with other kids who were equally as bored, or we would find sticks and draw countless illustrations in the dirt around the ballfield and parking lot. We were creative, used our imagination, and moved to keep entertained. Not a single kid could sit still through an entire baseball game, so we met up with new kids, introduced ourselves, played, and moved.

The way kids move is thought-provoking, and if you think about it, that flexibility is something most adults lose as they get older. Have you ever watched a toddler or young child playing on the ground? It's fascinating how effortlessly they can sit on the ground or squat down with their butt below their knees, drawing in the dirt or playing with a toy. This flexibility in young children is not only impressive but also a sign of good health in adults. It is something we need to maintain as we get older. Sitting on the ground or squatting low offers numerous benefits: it improves posture, aids digestion and circulation, enhances hip flexibility, relieves tension, and boosts overall mobility. Unfortunately, as we age, we often lose these simple abilities. You are never too old to play like a child, so join your children or grandchildren on the floor. Squat down and connect in playtime with them; build a castle, assemble LEGOs, or solve a puzzle together. Research even suggests that adults who can perform the sitting-rising test (rising from the floor without using their hands) tend to live longer, possibly by up to 10 years. So, get down on the ground and play!

If your kids participate in any sports, spend time outdoors with them, helping them practice and improve their skills. If they're involved in band or music, join them in playing instruments or singing and organizing at-home concerts to keep their passion alive. Sit at the kitchen table and color together. Encourage your kids to explore the kitchen by assigning them a meal to cook for the family. Cooking is a lifelong skill that they'll carry with them forever. It's also an excellent way to integrate various aspects of their education, from reading recipes and measuring ingredients to following instructions and creating something everyone can enjoy.

While microwaves and dishwashers may streamline mealtimes,

there's something special about cooking homemade meals and spending quality time in the kitchen together as a family (or even with friends). Go out to eat less often, order fewer take-out meals, and choose to create more home-cooked meals. Hiring a housecleaner or lawn service is convenient, and having groceries delivered or grabbing ready-made meals can save time. However, instead of paying to have these chores done, consider doing them yourself. Chores give us an opportunity to incorporate exercise into our daily routine. They also provide a chance to connect with friends and family, teach valuable lessons to our children, and reduce time spent with electronics.

Turning chores into enjoyable activities and doing them with loved ones can transform the work into something more enjoyable and promotes teamwork, which is beneficial as we enter the workforce. Collaborate to strengthen relationships with the people around you and add fun to the task at hand. Shift your perspective to appreciate your body's capabilities, whether you're hunting for asparagus, raking leaves, tackling landscaping projects, gardening, playing with your kids, or cooking in the kitchen. Discover the rewards in your chores.

I admit, when we were young, the small chores were not always enjoyable, but they gave us responsibility. Daily chores (like doing dishes) could be tedious. And, when all four of us girls wanted something "big," like a tire swing or a treehouse, we were asked to put in our own sweat equity to make it happen. The reward was found in a job well done.

Working alongside Mom or Dad to complete these larger and less monotonous tasks instilled in us a valuable lesson; we never took for granted that things would be done for us. Our efforts taught us resilience and determination, and when the job was complete, we felt a great sense of satisfaction. Chores are more than just tasks; they are a source of pride and accomplishment.

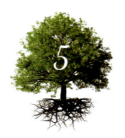

Nourishing Wellness:
The Power of Food and Nutrition

Mom and Dad were both good cooks. Both had areas of expertise that provided a good balance when it came to the meals we ate. Most of the time there were no written recipes required. The makings for a good meal were either all stored in memory or created in the moment with whatever ingredients were accessible. One night, I remember Dad making homemade scalloped potatoes and ham. The potatoes were, of course, from his garden, and the ham was from one of eight or so pigs he raised each year. I am not sure where Mom was that night, but she was not home, and my sisters gobbled up Dad's culinary creation and were excused from the table once their plates were clean. At the time, I was not a fan of scalloped potatoes, and to this day still do not care for mashed potatoes at all. Regardless, I was having trouble finishing the helping of white mush Dad dished up for me that night. I sat at the table alone, attempting to take the last few bites while Dad was washing up the stove. I just could not finish eating the homemade dish, so I decided to squish the remaining potatoes with my fork into a very thin mashed layer on the bottom of my plate to make it look like I had finished the meal. I figured that he would never know the difference. When Dad returned to the kitchen table to check on my progress, he did not buy into the notion that my plate was clean. He told me to get up from the table if I was done and then kindly warned me that I would get nothing else to eat that night if I was still hungry.

When Mom or Dad made a meal for the family, that one meal was what was being served. There were no alternatives. Mom and Dad did not rush to the stove to make a separate dish for a whiney child or grab a microwave dinner as a substitute because one of us (me) did not particularly like scalloped potatoes and ham. If any of us girls did not like what was being served, it was simply too bad. What was made that night for dinner would be served up as leftovers later that night if you got hungry. Now, that did not happen all that often because we were raised to eat whatever was made for us with no argument and truly learned to love most of the meals made for us. We grew up experiencing dishes like ham and bean soup, pork butt and cooked carrots, and deer roast and potatoes; dishes many kids today would make faces at and not even have the courage or curiosity to touch. Even in the instances when one of us did not want to eat what was served, none of us ever starved to death.

Food was straightforward back then. The ingredients were basic; the meals were simple. Options were limited too; often, there was just one choice. Nowadays, so many people complain about not having enough time to cook for themselves, let alone their families. People rely too much on quick and easy prepackaged or processed meals, or have premade food delivered to save time and effort on what they're putting into their bodies. Yet, when people do decide to make a meal for the entire family, they are juggling macaroni and cheese for the kids, a burger for Dad, and a salad for Mom's diet, which in turn results in a significant amount of time for just one meal (or multiple meals to appease all family members). No wonder making food for a family takes so much time!

Food is information. What we eat and drink molds every cell in our body, from the muscles of our heart to the tissue in our lungs to our bones and blood vessels. Our nutrition designs us! The body replaces 1% of our cells daily, which is roughly 330 BILLION cells! What we put in our mouths and consume literally changes the expression of our DNA, which is incredible. Every single one of us has tremendous power and control in how we continually develop through the foods we eat. We are what we eat!

> ❝ *Let food be thy medicine and medicine be thy food.*
> —Hippocrates, Father of Medicine

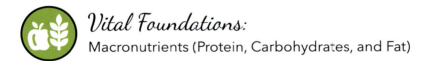

Vital Foundations: Macronutrients (Protein, Carbohydrates, and Fat)

THE POWER OF PROTEIN: Meat & More

Protein was always part of every meal. Our family enjoyed meat-based dishes. If we were not eating deer or pheasant, we were eating chicken, pork, or beef. Sometimes, we would have fish if it was available from a weekend of fishing at a nearby lake. Protein is a key component of our metabolic health. We need natural protein sources to build and retain muscle. Protein is the building block of healthy muscle, which is valuable real estate and becomes more precious to us as we age. Protein is the most important macronutrient humans consume, and there is a good reason for it.

In my high school days, athletes and busy parents were not loading up on protein powders and supplements. They really did not exist back then, and we did just fine. We ate plenty of protein in meat, dairy, nuts, beans, and certain vegetables. There was no need to supplement our diets with expensive protein shakes and protein bars. Today, the protein supplement market in the United States is over $10 billion.[1] Almost every brand uses a bold font on their labels that signifies strength, along with imagery of bigger muscles and a leaner physique. And almost every "powder" on the market is comprised of ingredients that might cause more harm than good, including preservatives to lengthen shelf life, artificial flavors, and fake sugars such as sucralose, dextrose, and aspartame.

The Mayo Clinic even states that, as long as you're eating a healthy diet, "you likely do not need to add extra protein through protein shakes or other sources." And most doctors say that incorporating protein supplements in your diet with no workout at all is not recommended. If you are an athlete and simply cannot consume enough calories and/or protein to sustain optimal weight and athletic performance, you might need a protein supplement. And that is okay, but please take the time to research quality protein supplements if you need one, in addition to looking at modifying your daily diet using real food.

With a careful selection of quality protein sources and real nutrients, it's entirely possible to meet your daily protein needs through whole foods. Eggs, plain Greek yogurt, cottage cheese, nut butters, nuts, and beans are excellent sources of protein. Additionally, a 4 oz serving of various meats provides significant protein: chicken (27g), beef (23g), salmon (24g), pork (24g), and turkey (23g). As omnivores, humans naturally thrive on a balanced diet including meat. So, why not fire up the grill and enjoy some steaks?

HORMONES AND ANTIBIOTICS in our Meat and Dairy Supply

Did you know that through the dairy and meat products we eat, we consume more hormones and antibiotics than we realize? Nearly all the meat that we buy at the grocery store comes from sources that are raised in large confinements in mass production. Animals who are raised in these confinements are fed a mixture of grain and feed, which really could be considered processed food for animals. Large amounts of grain are not a natural diet for cows, nor is it natural for cows to live in close quarters with no way of distancing themselves from their own manure.

Livestock confinements are not a pleasant way for animals of any kind to be raised. The definition of confinement is *captivity, immurement, imprisonment, incarceration, or the state of being imprisoned.* Whether it's cattle, hogs, chickens, or even turkeys, animals were not meant to consume manufactured feed or live in unsanitary conditions. Just drive by any animal confinement, and I am sure you will smell what I am talking about. Animals raised in confinements often require medications and antibiotics to prevent infections and illness. These animals are also given hormones to increase meat production. The bigger the animal and the faster they grow, the more they are worth. So, the confined animals eat their food products, including any hormones, antibiotics, and other medications that might be given to them or mixed in with their feed—and we eat these animals that have been pumped full of God-knows-what. Therefore, we are consuming not just the meat or dairy from these animals, but we are consuming everything that has been added to (not by nature) for those meat and dairy products. Remember, we are what we eat. And the animals we eat are what *they* eat.

When I was starting a family of my own in the early 2000s, Dad brought me a page of handwritten notes that he took while he was at work one day at the grain elevator. This page listed the hormones, antibiotics, and other drugs that get mixed into cattle feed, hog feed, and chicken feed to keep livestock "healthy." Dad wanted to explain to me what was being pumped into the meats typically found at the grocery store and why he chose to raise his own chickens and hogs for our family to eat. He did not want us to eat what he witnessed being fed to our food supply. He saw it firsthand at his job.

Dad would raise six to eight pigs every year. They would have the freedom to roam outside when they wanted with the option for shelter through a little door that took them inside the outbuilding we called the chicken house. The chickens also had the freedom to go outdoors to pick at the ground and eat bugs and worms. The pigs (and chickens) got fed leftovers from our meals, rotten vegetables and fruits from our gardens, melon rinds, and empty cobs of sweet corn. When one of Dad's pigs got sick, he would care for the animal the best he could and attempt to make it well. But if the pig was too sick and died, that was life. There was no pumping it full of medications to try and save it; it would die, and it would be one less pig that Dad would take to butcher. His philosophy was, "You don't want to eat sick meat." That made sense to me.

It was important to Dad that we ate "clean" meat. After all those years working at the grain elevator and mixing feed for farmers, Dad knew what was going into the food the animals were eating. He wanted to keep his daughters (and grandchildren) from being exposed to what he claimed was poisonous. Dad told me that he had to wear gloves and a mask when working with these substances at the elevator before mixing them into the feed that he would deliver to farms. He also went on to tell me stories about how he witnessed hogs so frantic and hyped up on "speed" when they were being loaded into trailers that they would die of a heart attack right there on the loading ramp. They would go to slaughter anyway and be sold

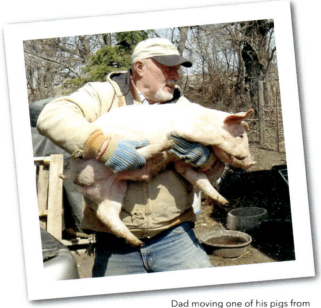

Dad moving one of his pigs from the truck into the chicken house.

for consumption. He referred to the handwritten list he gave me and said it was basically a combination of steroids and speed to get the animals to grow bigger and faster along with antibiotics and medications to keep them from getting sick and dying from living in filthy conditions. More meat, more money!

After researching each one of the ingredients listed on that piece of paper that Dad gave me, I quickly found out that most of them are banned in other countries.

Go with grass-fed organic beef and dairy and free-range chicken and eggs.

Basic BLT on Sourdough

2 slices Sourdough Bread, lightly toasted
3-4 slices thick-cut Bacon, cooked until crispy
2 leaves Romaine Lettuce
1 ripe garden Tomato, sliced
1-2 tablespoon(s) Mayonnaise
1/2 Avocado, sliced (optional)

Lightly toast the sourdough bread until golden. Spread a thin layer of mayonnaise on one or both slices. Layer the romaine lettuce, tomato slices, and crispy bacon on one slice of bread. To make the sandwich extra creamy, add sliced avocado. Top with the second slice of bread and slice in half.

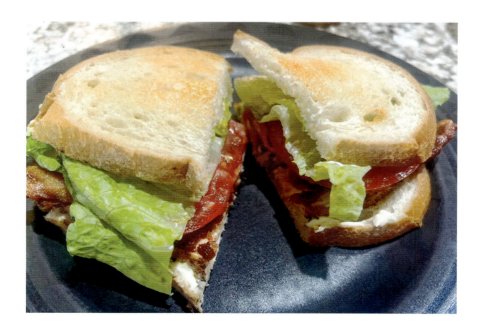

Grilled Iowa Pork Chops

4 one-inch-thick Iowa Pork Chops
Sea Salt and ground Black Pepper
Optional sides: Asparagus, Broccoli, and/or Brown Rice

Heat the grill to 325 degrees. Season the chops with salt and pepper. Lay the meat on the grill and let cook for about 8 to 10 minutes on each side. When the internal temperature reaches 145 degrees, they are ready to eat. You can also pan-fry chops in a cast iron skillet on the stove, browning the chops on both sides. If your chops are lean, you might decide to add a bit of olive oil or bacon grease to the pan to keep the meat from sticking to it. Serve with roasted broccoli, grilled asparagus, or a side of brown rice.

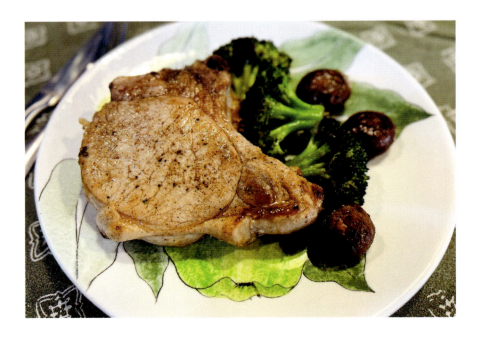

Low-Carb, No-Carb, or Carb UP?

Carbohydrates are considered energy, and most of the carbs our family ate (and still do) come from plants—colorful garden vegetables. Starchier plants like potatoes, yams, and squash I refer to as "ground carbs." These are complex carbohydrates and take longer to digest (complex to digest), leaving you feeling fuller longer. Complex carbs are full of vitamins, nutrients, prebiotics, and probiotics. These are the "good carbs" full of fiber. Mandate vegetables!

Bread, pasta, and rice were also part of our diet growing up. These are considered simple carbs (quick energy) and are typically already processed and take less effort for our digestive systems to work (simple to digest). Homemade breads are much different and much better for you than the white bread you find on the grocery store shelves. Processed simple carbs typically come in a box or package: granola bars, cereal, crackers, snack cakes, cookies, ice cream, soda…these can be "bad carbs" and are easy to digest, leaving you feeling hungry soon after a meal and then only craving more of the bad carbs. Because they are so simple to digest, they can also give you a spike in glucose (sugar). Frequent spikes in glucose can result in insulin resistance, which is a precursor to type 2 diabetes.

Mom was and still is to this day a fabulous bread maker! There is nothing like warm slices of home-baked bread straight out of the oven with real butter and maybe even a little touch of local honey. When Mom would make bread, she did it in bulk and would double-wrap and freeze several loaves for us to enjoy at a later date. This would save her time by baking in large quantities. Mom's homemade bread consisted of water, flour, oil, yeast, sugar, and salt. Six ingredients; the basics. Store-bought bread can contain up to twenty-five ingredients, most of which you cannot even pronounce. Homemade bread will mold within a week. Store-bought bread with all the ingredients

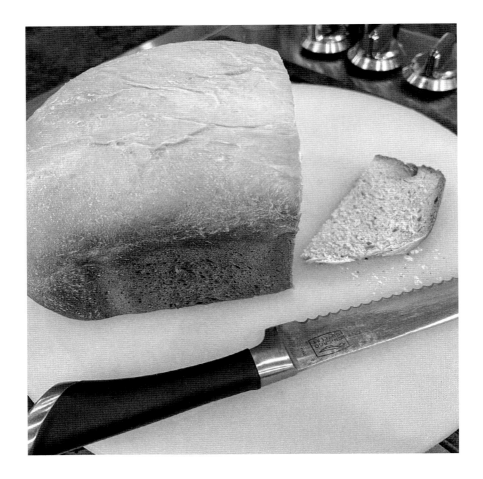

in it will last several weeks, even months. If it takes that long for it to decompose, why would we eat it?

We need carbohydrates (good carbohydrates) to live and function optimally. They are our main source of fuel, and our bodies and brains need good carbohydrates to operate efficiently. But not all carbs are created equal. Complex carbs are better than simple carbs, and unadulterated sources are best. Pure sources of carbohydrates have one ingredient like potatoes, spinach, apples, strawberries, and yams. When carbohydrates are manufactured (produced in a factory), nutrients are often stripped away, and preservatives are added. If you need to buy prepackaged carbs from the grocery store, choose baked goods with the shortest ingredient list—fewer additives mean healthier options. And the ingredients in those products should be ones you can pronounce and ones you would typically find in your pantry at home.

When I was in college, the Atkins diet was popular. Today, the Keto diet has taken its place. Neither one of these diet trends is bad, but when you eliminate carbohydrates from the typical American diet, with most of the carbs consumed being highly processed carbs full of sugar and unrecognizable ingredients, you are bound to lose weight. When you eliminate processed (unrecognizable) foods from your diet and replace them with more natural options, you are unsurprisingly going to use the nutrients from what you are eating and digest what your body does not need from those foods more efficiently.

Enjoy a healthy slice of sourdough or French baguette bread or dig into a bowl of quality pasta. Just make sure that your serving sizes are the recommended serving size. Bread is usually one slice, or pasta might be one cup, not three. And, when you are enjoying a good pasta dish make sure that your sauce is rich in protein and vegetables. Use less pasta (carbs) and more meat (protein) and vegetables such as spinach and mushrooms. The sauce is the tastiest part of the dish anyway. There is no need to eliminate carbs altogether. Bon Appetit!

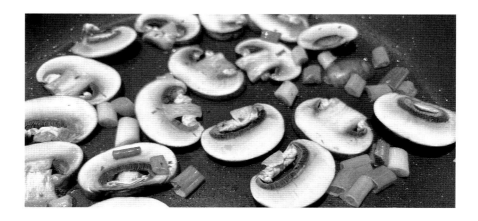

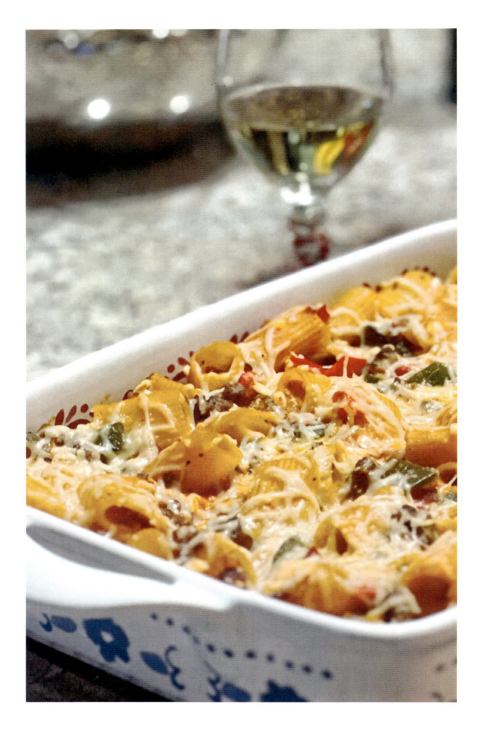

Hull of a Pasta Dish

1 lb. of Ziti noodles
1-1/2 lbs. Ground Italian Sausage
1 cup of Cottage Cheese
1 jar of "low sugar" Marinara Sauce
1 chopped Purple Onion
2 cups of Spinach Leaves
2 chopped Tomatoes
2 teaspoon Garlic Salt
2 teaspoon Basil
1 cup shredded Mozzarella
1/2 cup shredded Parmesan
Tomato slices & Basil leaves to decorate the top

Place the noodles in a pot of water and boil. Brown the sausage in a large skillet while the noodles are boiling. Once the meat is brown, add the spinach, onion, tomatoes, and spices. Stir until spinach leaves wilt. Drain the noodles once al dente. Mix pasta, meat & veggies, a jar of marinara (watch the sugar content), and cottage cheese in a bowl. Pour the mixture into a large baking dish. Top with shredded cheese and decorate the top of your casserole with sliced tomatoes and basil leaves. Cover and bake at 375°F for 35 minutes.

Roasted Roots

4 whole Carrots

4 whole Parsnips (peeled)

2 Sweet Potatoes (peeled and quartered)

2 Potatoes (quartered, skins on)

Carbs from the ground are the best carbs. Wash the dirt off your vegetables. Peel the parsnips and sweet potatoes. Quarter the sweet potatoes and potatoes longways. Place your "ground carbs" on a cookie sheet. Drizzle with olive oil and add a bit of sea salt. Drizzle a touch of local honey over the parsnips and sweet potatoes. Bake for 40 minutes (or until tender) at 375°F.

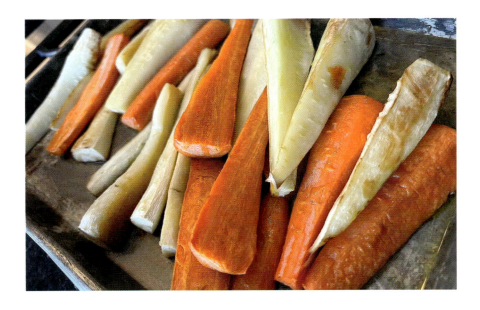

Fat-Free, Low-Fat, or Full-Fat?

Fat is good. We need fat! Yes, I said it! The fat-free, low-fat craze did us more harm than good. 80% of the United States population does not get enough essential fatty acids in their diet. Fats (healthy omegas) are important for the absorption of vitamins, brain function, and healthy skin and hair. Fats provide energy, help reduce inflammation and produce hormones. Lack of fats in our diet can lead to constipation, gallstones, and premature aging. Healthy fats that come from animals (meat and dairy) are good for us. Healthy fats that come from plants (olives, avocados, and nuts) are good for us; that is why they are called essential fatty acids.

Dad loved to grill, and whenever he grilled steak or pork chops, we girls would typically trim the fat from our cuts of meat. Dad would always tell us to eat the fat; it was good for us. He always ate the fat on his meat and sometimes would even finish the scraps from our plates (even the gristle). Dad also loved eating chicken tails! Yes, the little triangle piece of fatty flesh from the chicken's backside that its tail feathers were once connected to. Chicken tails are nothing but a chunk of fat, and Dad would gobble them up! We would always save the tail for Dad, and every time he put one into his mouth and started to chew, we would cringe. Despite all the fat Dad ate, his cholesterol and blood pressure levels were always healthy.

There are good fats, and there are bad fats. Factory-made fats like vegetable oils, soybean oils, and seed oils undergo a lengthy process, starting with the crushing of large seeds, followed by heating and pressing for oil extraction. While this may not seem harmful initially, the oil is further processed through bleaching and deodorizing, leading to rancidity. So please avoid all seed oils and margarines. They are far from any natural sources of fat, and I could argue that they are foreign substances that our bodies do not recognize at all, disrupting normal bodily processes. They make us sick.

Choose unrefined extra-virgin olive oil for cooking. Coconut oil and avocado oil are also excellent options too. These oils are extracted simply by squeezing the fruit they come from without undergoing bleaching or deodorizing processes. Simple, basic, and better for our bodies.

Eat real butter, full-fat plain Greek yogurt, 4% cottage cheese, and whole milk. In addition to numerous health benefits, healthy fats are more filling and enhance the flavor of food. Extra virgin olive oil is also a great source of essential fatty acids. Simply add a sprinkle of Parmesan and red pepper flakes (or freshly ground black pepper) to the oil, then dip your Italian or French bread for a delicious treat.

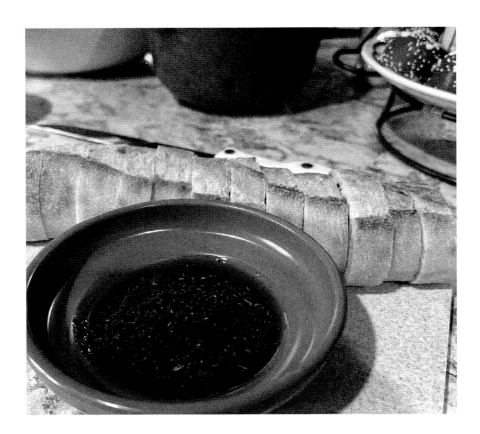

Omega Guacamole

2 ripe Avocados
2 Green Onions chopped
½ Jalapeno chopped
1 Lime squeezed
2 tablespoon chopped Cilantro (optional)
Sea Salt to taste

Avocados are healthy plant-based omegas. Cut them in half and remove the pit (save one pit). Scoop out the avocado meat, place it in a mixing bowl, and mash. Add the chopped onions and jalapeno along with the lime, cilantro, and sea salt. Stir well and serve with your favorite tortilla chips or use to top tacos or taco salad! If you have leftover guacamole, stir in a splash of vinegar. Place the leftover guacamole along with the saved pit in the refrigerator. The vinegar and avocado pit will keep your guacamole greener longer.

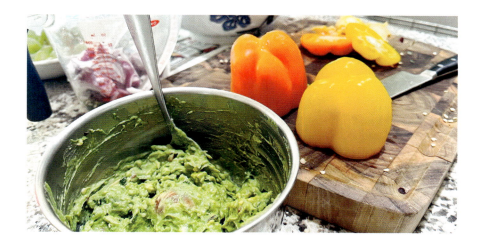

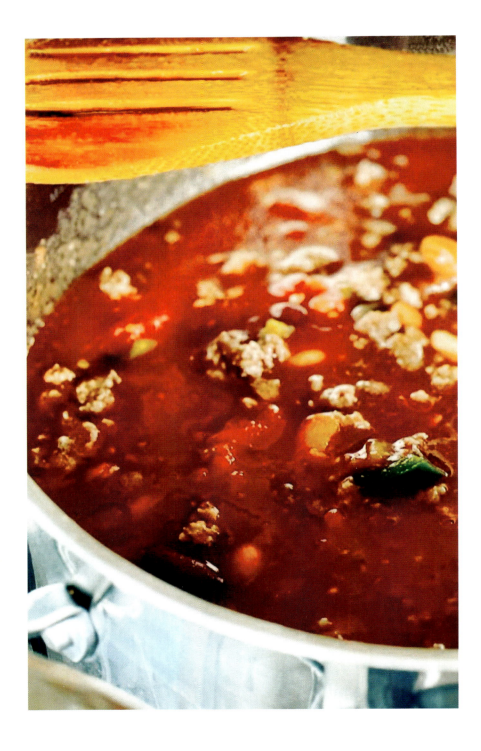

Protein-Packed Chili

1-1/2 lbs. Ground Beef
1 chopped White Onion
1 chopped Green Pepper
½ - 1 chopped Jalapeño
One 15.5 oz can of Red Kidney Beans
One 15.5 oz can of Navy Beans
One 15.5 oz can of Pinto Beans
Two 29oz cans of Diced Tomatoes
One 29oz can of Tomato Sauce
One can of Corn (optional)
2 Tablespoons Chili Powder

All healthy macronutrients can be found in this homemade chili. Plus, there are usually plenty of leftovers, which saves time in preparing healthy home-cooked meals later in a busy week. Brown the ground beef in a pan. Add the chopped onion and jalapeno and sauté for a few minutes to flavor the beef. Put all ingredients into either a large soup pan on the stove (low/medium heat) or slow cook crockpot and stir well. Let the chili heat and simmer. Stir occasionally and serve when hot. No seasoning packets or extra MSG is needed as chili is easily seasoned with natural ingredients. You can even create your own tomato sauce for chili with tomatoes fresh out of the garden.

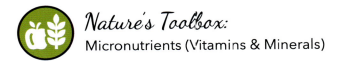

Nature's Toolbox:
Micronutrients (Vitamins & Minerals)

Vitamins and minerals are micronutrients needed to fight infections, build a strong immune system, and absorb macronutrients. We need them for optimum function. For example, vitamin C and the mineral zinc help us fight colds, while vitamin D and calcium help build strong bones. We can find plenty of pure micronutrients in the foods we eat, primarily natural foods.

We can also find micronutrients in supplements. And the supplements (which can be expensive) are just that—to supplement your nutrition and fill the gaps that you are not getting with real food. Consumers need to know that the Food and Drug Administration (FDA) does not pre-approve dietary supplements for safety, effectiveness, or labeling before they are made available to the public. It is the responsibility of dietary supplement companies to ensure that their products are safe and accurately labeled. Many supplements contain synthetic ingredients, flavors, dyes, and added sugar. In fact, some popular vitamin chews have more sugar in them than a piece of candy! If you can get your micronutrients from real food, it is probably a safer bet and will save you some money too.

Food manufacturers have been good at adding vitamins and minerals to their products. They proudly promote it, so consumers feel good buying and consuming them. Words like "refined," "enriched," and "fortified" all sound reliable, but know that those words are basically a way of saying that food has been "tampered with." Natural nutrients are often removed and replaced with synthetic ingredients in an attempt to reintroduce micronutrients into the processed food products being manufactured and sold. Synthetic flavors and colors are typically also added to enhance the flavor and appearance, most of which are harmful (and even hazardous) for long-term human consumption. Examples:

- **Allura Red AC** (aka Red 40) is a food coloring typically used in breakfast cereals. It is a synthetic red dye that is believed to cause hyperactivity and attention deficit disorder (ADD) in children when combined with sodium benzoate (a preservative). Red 40 is also believed to cause allergic reactions like hives and eczema. The FDA has approved this common ingredient for cosmetics, drugs, and foods; foods that we promote to young children. In Europe Red 40 is not recommended for children; in fact, it is banned in several European countries. Note: The U.S. recently banned Red No. 3 (announced January 15, 2025) giving food manufacturers until January 2027 and drug manufacturers until January 2028 to comply.

- **Folic Acid** is 100% synthetic (artificially made), and it is on everything. There is no natural nutrient called folic acid. Methylfolate (folate) is the natural nutrient found in green leafy vegetables, citrus fruit, and beans that helps facilitate the synthesis of the neurotransmitters associated with mood regulation. In 1998, the FDA required that synthetic folic acid be added to "enriched" cereal and grain products to reduce the risk of neural tube defects. 44% of the population cannot break down folic acid, which again is a synthetic/artificially made product. The side effects of folic acid are stomach upset, bloating, nausea, diarrhea, irritability, confusion, behavior changes, skin reactions, seizures, sleep pattern disturbance, etc. Foods labeled "enriched" or "fortified" have been sprayed with folic acid. All grains in the United States are sprayed with folic acid unless it is certified organic.

Unfortunately, the list goes on and on.

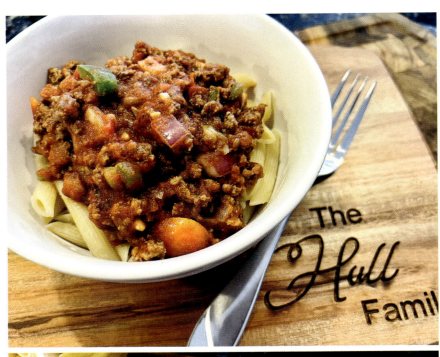
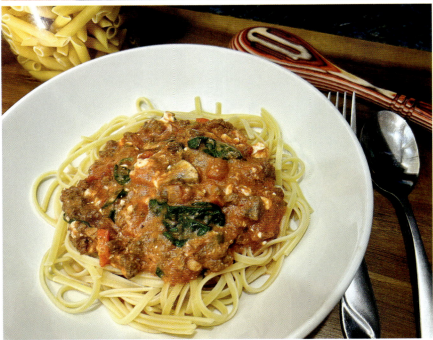

Vitamin Rich Pasta Sauce

- **1 lb of Ground Beef, Italian Sausage or Ground Turkey**
- **1 jar of Marinara Sauce (store-bought or homemade)**
- **2 cups of chopped Veggies (Mushrooms, Onions, Tomatoes, Peppers, Zucchini…)**
- **1 cup Cottage Cheese (optional for creamier sauce and extra protein)**

Chop a variety of colorful vegetables of your choice. Get creative and use various combinations. Brown the meat in a large pan. Once the meat is fully cooked, add the 2 cups of vegetables to the pan and sauté them with the meat until bright and tender. Pour the marinara sauce into the pan. Heat and serve over 1 cup of your favorite pasta noodles. If you choose to go meatless; heat 1-2 tablespoon(s) of extra virgin olive oil in a large saucepan. Add the 2 cups of vegetables to the pan and sauté until tender. Pour the marinara sauce over the sautéed vegetables, add the cottage cheese (optional for a meatless protein source), stir and heat well. Once the pan of sauce is hot, your vitamin rich sauce is ready to serve.

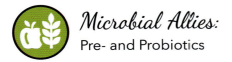

Microbial Allies:
Pre- and Probiotics

Our gut hosts up to 100 trillion microorganisms that are important to our overall health. This collection of microorganisms is called the microbiome and includes bacteria, viruses, fungi, and other microbes that live in and on the human body, particularly in the digestive tract, skin, mouth, and other mucosal surfaces. Our microbiome plays a crucial role in various physiological processes, including digestion, immune function, metabolism, and even mental health. Your microbiome (gut health) is directly affected by diet, lifestyle, genetics, and environmental exposures.

Prebiotics and probiotics are both used to promote gut health, but they serve different functions. Prebiotics are non-digestible fibers found in certain foods, such as fruits, vegetables, whole grains, and legumes. They act as food for beneficial bacteria in the gut, helping them to grow and thrive. Probiotics are live microorganisms, usually bacteria or yeasts, which are found in certain foods (like yogurt, kefir, and fermented vegetables) and dietary supplements. Both prebiotics and probiotics help maintain a healthy balance of gut microbiota, which aid in digestion, support immune function, reduce inflammation, and ease symptoms of certain digestive disorders.

The prebiotics and probiotics market in the United States is over $60 billion in annual sales! There is a reason for it; people can't poop. Consumers have destroyed their gut microbiome by overconsuming ultra-processed foods and failing to include enough natural, whole foods in their diet. People are constipated! The average American's diet is 60-70% processed food. And it is not just adults; the same statistics can be applied to our children too. Eating more natural foods and less ultra-processed foods is an easy way to get more prebiotics and probiotics naturally in our diet, improving our microbiome without having to spend a ton on supplements that claim they promote gut health.

Like most dietary supplements, pre- and probiotics do not require FDA approval unless they make health claims. So read your labels, make sure the ingredients are pure, and spend your money wisely. Supplements can be very expensive, and most of the time, we can get our vitamins, minerals, and prebiotics/probiotics by consuming real food.

A diverse gut is a healthy gut. Eat a variety of real foods!

Whole Lot of Goodness Yogurt Parfait

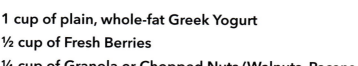

1 cup of plain, whole-fat Greek Yogurt
½ cup of Fresh Berries
¼ cup of Granola or Chopped Nuts (Walnuts, Pecans, and/or Almonds)

Scoop yogurt into a bowl. Top with fresh berries of your choice and granola and/or chopped nuts. Enjoy!

Tip: yogurt parfaits are easy to make ahead of time and pack for school or work lunches. They are not only great for breakfast but also serve as a good afternoon snack!

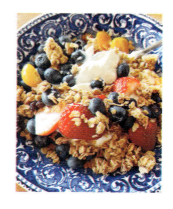

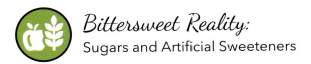

Bittersweet Reality:
Sugars and Artificial Sweeteners

Before Dad got his job at the grain elevator (the Fenton Co-op), he worked at Snap-On Tools in Algona, Iowa. He had the night shift and would get home early in the morning. On the occasional Saturday morning after his Friday overnight shift, he would stop at a convenience store (aka gas station) and pick up a six-pack of packaged donuts; two powdered sugar, two cinnamon, and two plain. They came in a white rectangle box with a see-through cellophane top. There were just enough in the box for each of us to have just one. Donuts were a treat. Dad only brought them home once in a great while. The four of us girls could not wait to wake up on Saturday mornings to see if it was a donut day. We were up earlier on Saturday mornings than we were for school Monday through Friday for three reasons: 1) we would get to have breakfast with Dad, 2) we would sometimes get surprised with donuts for breakfast, and 3) we got to watch Saturday morning cartoons.

Dad also, on occasion, would allow us to buy soda pop, Shasta to be exact. Shasta soda pop was an off-brand, unlike the more popular Pepsi or Coke. It came in all different flavors and brightly colored cans that coincided with the contents inside. Shasta was only ten cents for each twelve-ounce can, which was a bargain (even back then). So, every now and then when we all went to the grocery store as a family, Dad would give us each permission to pick out two to three cans each from a huge bin by the check-out lines at the front of the grocery store. He happily bought sodas for all his girls for just over a dollar. My favorite flavor was cream soda, probably because it was Dad's favorite. He also liked root beer and would occasionally add a scoop of vanilla ice cream to it for a frothy root beer float. My three younger sisters liked the fruit-flavored Shasta. I am sure the bright-colored cans influenced their selections like most kids.

We also loved Kool-Aid! Remember the Kool-Aid Man; how he would break through walls in 1980s TV commercials shouting, "Ohhh Yeah!" Whacky wild Kool-Aid style was making your own soft drink mix at home with 3 packets of your favorite flavor (or color) Kool-Aid drink powders, one gallon of water, and 1 ½ cups of white sugar! So much sugar, and we would drink that stuff by the gallons!

Other than the occasional donut, can of soda, or big glass of Kool-Aid, our family stuck to the essentials. Mom even stuck with the basics when it came to breakfast cereal. When most kids our age were eating "fun" and sugar-coated cereals that were advertised during Saturday morning cartoons like Captain Crunch, Frosted Flakes, Lucky Charms, and Cocoa Puffs, we were stuck with Wheaties, Corn Flakes, Shredded Wheat, and plain Cheerios. No cartoon character on the box, no extra sugars, no fancy colors, and definitely no marshmallows.

When it came to desserts, the only time we got them was when Mom would sporadically make homemade cookies or around the holidays when she would bake homemade pie. Mom made the best pies that consisted of Grandma Nita's homemade crust recipe and usually apples from our apple trees. The crust was the absolute best and was made from scratch with good old-fashioned Crisco, flour, water, and salt. Mom would intentionally make a generous amount of dough, ensuring there were plenty of scraps from trimming the excess that extended beyond the pie plate. Mom would take the scraps "as is" in their various shapes and sizes, lay them on a cookie sheet, sprinkle them with sugar and cinnamon, and stick them in the oven. Mom called these delicious pie crust scraps "crispies." They didn't take long to bake—maybe five to ten minutes—and as soon as we girls caught the warm, sweet scent of cinnamon wafting upstairs to our bedrooms, we'd come running down the stairs into the kitchen to claim our "crispy" from the hot cookie sheet. Crispies were our favorite. I always tried to be the first in the kitchen to grab the biggest one.

Birthday cakes were also a big deal at the Brink house. They were not always pretty, but they were always homemade and delicious. Mom's cold water chocolate cake was to die for. Usually, all our birthday cakes were accompanied by ice cream from the store, which we had on hand for more than just birthdays, and to satisfy Dad's occasional craving for a root beer float or bowl of ice cream topped with cashews and chocolate syrup.

Desserts were not a daily treat; they were meant to be a sometimes food and only intended to be had once in a great while and for special occasions like birthdays and holidays. Dessert was a luxury. Today, dessert has become a staple at nearly every meal, and many breakfasts are actually dessert-like food (muffins, sweet breads, sugary cereals, flavored coffees, etc.). Whether it is the cookies included

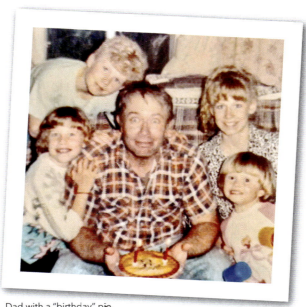

Dad with a "birthday" pie.

in school lunch menus, brownies that are part of a catered meal for work functions, or a slice of pie or cake that is served in retirement homes or hospitals, dessert is almost always present and has become a regular part of our daily diet.

Recent studies highlight the significant negative effects of consuming excessive amounts of added sugars, especially in children. Diets high in added sugars can impair immune function and contribute to systemic inflammation, potentially weakening the body's ability to fight infections. Additionally, excessive sugar intake is linked to cognitive issues, including memory and learning difficulties, due to its effects on brain health, such as increased oxidative stress and inflammation. The American Heart Association recommends that children consume no more than 25 grams of added sugar per day to reduce these risks and support overall health.[2]

Breakfast cereals are like dessert, and that is how most kids (and even adults) start their day; on empty calories with little to no real nutrients and a lot of added sugar. On top of starting their day with sweetened breakfast cereals, kids drink way too many sugary drinks like juice, soda, and even energy drinks. Chocolate and strawberry milk have become staples, while plain white milk is nearly a thing of the past. Sugar, sugar, and more sugar!

Sugar is a drug. Sugar is a white powder derived from a plant. Doesn't it sound like other drugs that come in a white, powdery form? Sugar affects the brain and is just as addictive as alcohol and tobacco. Eating sweets can make us feel happy or seemingly relieve tension and anxiety, which leads us to addiction.

There is "added sugar" in almost all ultra-processed foods (even in ketchup and spaghetti sauces). And if the label is bragging about "zero sugars," there are usually fake sugars to take sugar's place, which are almost worse than "real" sugar. Artificial sweeteners are 100-700x sweeter than real sugar and trick our brains into craving more sweets. The sweeter they are, the stronger our need for a dopamine fix that our brains want, and we start to rely on it to get us through the day. Fake sugars not only mess with our brains, but frequent use of these chemicals can create an imbalance in our gut bacteria. Artificial sweeteners are a sure way to sabotage our diet, and it is best to just steer clear of them altogether.

There is one living thing that not only loves sugar but thrives on it, cancer cells. Cancer cells are living cells that divide uncontrollably. Normal cells grow, divide, and eventually die, but not cancer cells. Cancer cells divide and produce other abnormal cells, and they feed off sugar; in fact, they love it. Cancer cells consume sugar at a rate 200x faster than normal cells! Think about it, PET-CT scans use a form of radioactive glucose (sugar) to activate where the body uses (eats) this form of sugar for testing. Cancer cells need this energy to grow, so when there is cancer present, the PET-CT scan will light up where cancer is in the body. Many cells in our bodies have the potential to turn into cancerous cells. For every additional 5g of sugar consumed in liquid form per day (think of your daily soda or coffee drink), cancer incidence increases by 8%. Why feed the cancer monster with added sugars in our diet?

I remember there would be times when my younger sisters would have either a pink, purple, or orange mustache from drinking fruit-flavored Shasta. Mom would wipe the stache from their faces with a wet washcloth to get the sticky off. Just like sugar leaves a sticky residue on our fingers, lips, and teeth, sugar can leave our insides literally sticky too. Think about sugar sticking to the insides of your small blood vessels! This further explains the negative effects sugar has on the human body.

Be sure to check labels for "added sugars." The average American consumes more than 68 grams of added sugar daily, which is equivalent to 17 teaspoons or more than 54 pounds of sugar each year. Children, on average, consume 81 grams per day, amounting to over 65 pounds annually. This amount is two to three times more than the recommended daily intake set by both the Dietary Guidelines for Americans and the World Health Organization.[3] To visualize this, the average American consumes between 13 and 20 four-pound bags of white sugar every year!

Ideally, we should limit sugar intake to 25g to 30g per day. Natural sugars found in fruit are okay. "Added sugars" are the ones you must watch out for. Watch out for common forms of added sugars in foods, including corn syrup, fructose, lactose, maltose, sucrose, dextrose, high fructose corn syrup, molasses, raw sugar, and table sugar.

When it comes to desserts (a sometimes treat, of course), nothing beats homemade! Forget the store-bought stuff—these recipes from my Grandma Nita's recipe box (and one from my Kindergarten cookbook) bring back wonderful memories, are fun to make, and even more delightful to share and enjoy with family and friends!

Banana Carrot Cake

½ C. Butter or margarine
¾ c. brown sugar - firmly packed
2 eggs
2 C flour   1 c. grated carrots
1 teas soda   ½ C - raisins
½ teas bkg. powder
½ teas cinnamon   350°
¼ teas salt   45 min
1 c mashed ripe bananas (3)

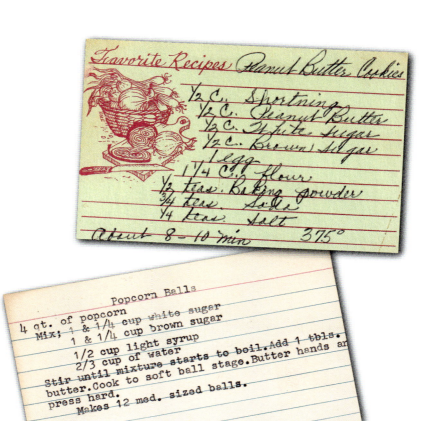

Favorite Recipes — Peanut Butter Cookies

½ C. Shortning
½ C. Peanut Butter
½ C. White Sugar
½ C. Brown Sugar
1 egg
1¼ C. flour
½ teas. Baking powder
¾ teas. Soda
¼ teas. Salt

About 8-10 min   375°

Popcorn Balls

4 qt. of popcorn
Mix; 1 & 1/4 cup white sugar
1 & 1/4 cup brown sugar
1/2 cup light syrup
2/3 cup of water
Stir until mixture starts to boil. Add 1 tbls. butter. Cook to soft ball stage. Butter hands and press hard.
Makes 12 med. sized balls.

Cherry Salad

1 Can sour cherries - drained
  not pie cherries
1 small Can Condensed Milk - blend in
2 tbls Lemon juice
1 small carton cool whip
1 small can pineapple tidbits

fold all together

NOURISHING WELLNESS

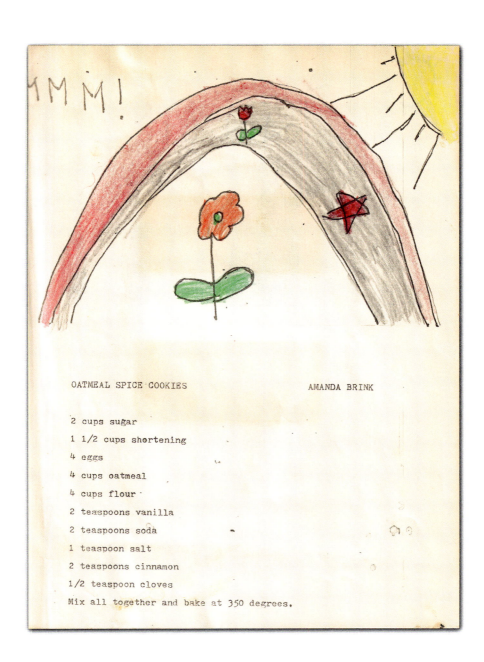

OATMEAL SPICE COOKIES   AMANDA BRINK

2 cups sugar

1 1/2 cups shortening

4 eggs

4 cups oatmeal

4 cups flour

2 teaspoons vanilla

2 teaspoons soda

1 teaspoon salt

2 teaspoons cinnamon

1/2 teaspoon cloves

Mix all together and bake at 350 degrees.

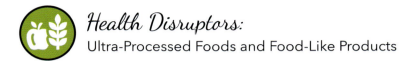

Health Disruptors:
Ultra-Processed Foods and Food-Like Products

One in eight children is addicted to ultra-processed foods, and there's a notable similarity between the addictive nature of these foods and substances like alcohol and tobacco.[4] Former tobacco giant Philip Morris shifted its focus to food, merging with Kraft-General Foods and Nabisco to produce popular brands such as Oreo, Ritz, Betty Crocker, and Oscar Mayer. Food companies employ tens of thousands of scientists to create food that is addictive and non-filling, heightening our cravings so we eat more. Eat more, buy more, eat more, buy more…The creation of these food-like substances is a calculated science that does not focus on nutrition but rather corporate greed. We are all being manipulated, and it has led to the obesity epidemic in America.

It is hard to avoid processed foods. The inside aisles of the grocery store are filled with bright bags and boxes and eye-catching packaging that lure you to factory-made options, which are less like actual food and more like food-like products. These processed foods are riddled with preservatives, chemicals, added sugars like high-fructose corn syrup, and other ingredients our bodies simply do not recognize.

Eat natural foods that you can find around the outside of the grocery store: fresh produce, eggs and dairy, meats, and fresh bakery goods. Shop the perimeter of the grocery store and avoid the inside aisles. Eating clean will make a huge difference in your overall health. Having your health is the ultimate convenience.

You should eat natural foods that decay and rot, rather than those filled with preservatives meant to prevent foods from spoiling. Consider a typical package of Twinkies or a block of Velveeta cheese.

Both can sit on store shelves for several months and even years without spoiling. The combination of preservatives, artificial flavorings, and high sugar content allows these processed foods to maintain their appealing texture and flavor for far longer than their natural counterparts, which would typically spoil much sooner. However, it's important to question what additives are used to prolong its freshness and how they may impact your health. When we consume foods with added preservatives and chemicals, we're essentially introducing foreign substances into our bodies. Processed foods result in allergies, obesity, and sickness.

In fact, preservatives were once called anti-digestives! Think about that for a minute...Preservatives and additives are added to factory foods to prolong shelf life and maintain a certain appearance. While these may keep the food looking fresh for an extended period, they often come at the cost of nutritional value and can introduce potentially harmful substances into our bodies. Anti-digest?

The "anti-digestives" found in our food have a direct impact on our digestive systems. Natural foods naturally decompose over time due to the absence of these preservatives. Although this may result in a shorter shelf life, it also implies they're generally devoid of artificial additives, contain more of their inherent nutrients, and are much easier on our digestive systems. Choose unprocessed foods without additives for better digestive health.

Like the jars of green beans Mom would can and the bags of frozen peas we would shuck, minimally processed and preserved foods are second best. Foods like canned or frozen fruits and vegetables consist of natural ingredients; no preservatives are needed, and they are minimally processed. Just watch for added MSG in canned vegetables and added sugars like high-fructose corn syrup in canned fruit.

Always read food labels, not necessarily for calories or fat content, but for the list of ingredients. If you cannot pronounce the ingredients, and the ingredients are not something you would find in your pantry at home, do not buy it and don't consume it. My theory is that if you cannot pronounce it, your body doesn't biologically recognize it.

Processed foods offer convenience, while preparing real food requires effort. Despite the allure of convenience, prioritizing health means considering better alternatives. There are natural foods (with only one ingredient) that are just as convenient as a bag of chips or a granola bar loaded with sugar to pack into lunchboxes or grab as a snack, such as a banana, an apple, strawberries, a handful of almonds, or dried fruit. Or take 20 minutes and make a dozen homemade peanut butter balls for the week, which are a well-balanced sweet treat that includes protein. These are great for breakfast on the go or an afternoon snack.

Be mindful about what you put into your body for nutrition. Be intentional about your health and wellness. Convenience can cost you your health. Invest in better food options and devote time to learning about better nutrition. Get back to basics. Consume simple and natural ingredients. It could save your life and bless you with more time here on this Earth.

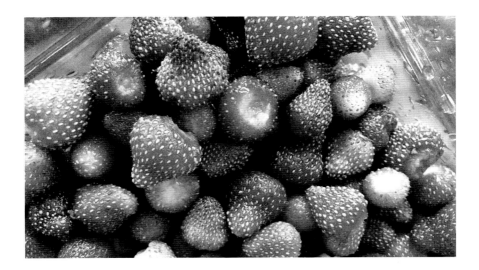

Oatmeal Peanut Butter Balls

- 2 cups Rolled Oats
- 2 cups Peanut, Almond, or Sun Butter
- ¼ cup mini Dark Chocolate Chips
- ¼ cup unsalted Sunflower Seeds
- 2 tablespoon Honey
- 2 tablespoon of Hemp, Flax, or Chia Seeds

Put all ingredients in a mixing bowl. Mix well and roll into 1 inch balls and chill.

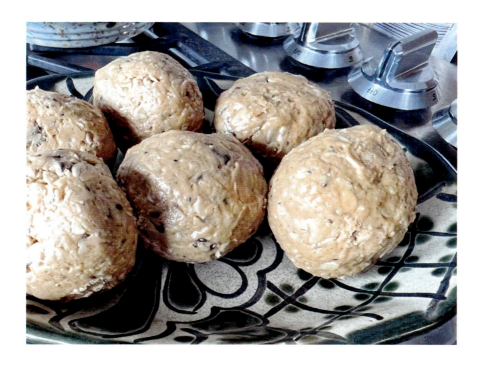

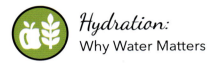

Hydration:
Why Water Matters

It is not just what we eat but what we drink that is important. Staying hydrated is super important and we should be drinking half an ounce to one full ounce of water for every pound we weigh. When we are dehydrated, the large intestine cannot provide enough water to properly form stools, which leads to constipation. Water makes up 60% of your body. It's important for healthy skin, hair, and nails, and helps to regulate body temperature, lubricate joints, flush waste, and reproduce cells.

Energy drinks are promoted as a great way to stay hydrated, but it's crucial to steer clear of all sugary beverages. This includes energy drinks and fruit juices, which are often loaded with as much sugar as the sodas—like Shasta—that my sisters and I drank during our childhood. Like most food companies, the labels and slogans leave you feeling like you need to drink them to perform well in sports and/or maintain energy throughout the day. Not true. Water can be just as good to stay hydrated, and if you are getting enough sodium, potassium, and chloride in your diet, you should not need to "supplement" your diet with energy drinks. Fruits, vegetables, meat, dairy, nuts, and whole grains are great sources of natural electrolytes.

Get your water in. But if you drink bottled water, be aware that the companies selling it aren't really selling water—they're selling plastic bottles. So, invest in a glass or stainless-steel water bottle and carry it with you everywhere. If plain water is not your jam and you need some flavor, add freshly squeezed lemon, slices of cucumber, mint leaves, or even cut-up strawberries.

You Are What You Eat...

Physique is 80% of the nutrition you consume, not necessarily how much you work out, although exercise is important too. People look at me and assume that I work out three to four hours a day—a gym rat. Not true. I work out one hour five days per week. My workouts consist of a walk with our dog and thirty to forty-five minutes of a "CrossFit" like workout. Mind you, I am also active outside of daily routine workouts, meaning I just move more throughout a typical day. I am well-toned and weigh 135 pounds (roughly the same weight I was in high school). Eating clean has a larger impact on appearance than hours spent in the gym. There is a saying, "You can't outrun your fork," and it is so true. The food we eat not only can determine how thin or fat we are, but it also determines our muscle tone and how good (or bad) our skin, hair, and nails look.

People are also amazed at the amount of food I eat. I do eat a lot, and it consists of mostly all natural foods; one ingredient, nothing processed or that comes from a factory. All calories are not created equal. Both meals outlined below are 350 calories. One will keep you feeling fuller longer, will promote healthy muscle and strong bones, has more nutrients, no added sugars, and no preservatives. I know which one I would rather eat. You?

Soda & Chips	Chicken, Broccoli & a Potato
(2 items. Over 30 ingredients)	(4 items. 4 ingredients)
12 oz soda ....150 calories	6 oz chicken ....150 calories
Nacho cheese chips ......200 calories	1-½ cup broccoli................40 calories
	1 small potato ....110 calories
	1 orange.............................50 calories
TOTAL: 350 calories	TOTAL: 350 calories

So, as you can see from the example above, not all calories are created equal. You can consume a greater quantity of good food for the same number of calories as an unhealthy snack. And, if you like to eat, why wouldn't you choose to eat more of the good stuff?

When my two kids were growing up, the rule at our house as far as snacks went was to eat as many fruits and vegetables as you wanted. If they wanted a snack outside of regular mealtime, they did not even need to ask permission. If they needed a little something between meals to tide them over, they could grab a piece of fruit or snack on fresh veggies. No limit: have as much as you want. There were many times when either one of them would devour an entire pint of blueberries or a half pound of grapes. Let's just say that they always pooped well!

And, just like Mom and Dad, I have always cooked a homemade meal every night for me and my family to ensure the quality of our nutrition. No matter how many hours I spent at work during my busy career, being home in time to make dinner, sit around the table with my family, and enjoy good nutrition together has always been a priority. You must make it one. My family has never consumed loads of microwave dinners and frozen pizzas. We enjoy real butter, whole milk, farm-fresh eggs, beef, pork, chicken, fish, and limitless amounts of fresh fruits and vegetables. The amount of soda and snack food is very limited and considered a treat.

Real food should be something to celebrate, and we should all embrace every opportunity to celebrate with food. It nourishes the body and brings people together. And, like family mealtimes, good food is a way to connect with others in social settings and makes for a great way to celebrate life with both family and friends. There is nothing better than sharing a beautiful meal with those you love and appreciate. Good nutrition is meant to be shared. If you have extra produce from your garden, a great recipe, or leftovers, share them.

Invite others to enjoy a home-cooked meal with you and pass on the gift of nutrition.

Both of my children learned to cook at an early age and were comfortable working in the kitchen ever since they could see over the countertop. Today, both are talented chefs making homemade pizzas, fettuccine noodles from scratch, chocolate chip cookies, and roasted vegetables. Cooking is a lifelong skill. So, if you have children, teach them to cook.

Experiment in the kitchen and have the courage to try new foods. You never know what you might be missing, and you could discover your new favorite food! I always tell people to "eat a rainbow of foods." The various colors of fruits and vegetables represent various antioxidants, which protect our cells from damage. Add more color to your plate. Not only is it eye appealing, but colors offer a variety of vitamins and minerals necessary for optimum health.

Always keep in mind that food serves as more than just nourishment; it's information for our bodies. It not only shapes how long we can live but how good we feel while living. By taking control of our nutrition, we can actively control our health and well-being. Eating a healthy diet is one way we can prevent, reverse, and improve many diseases. Take the time and invest in good nutrition. Prioritizing health through what we consume is not only a gift to ourselves but also to those around us.

There is more happiness in health than in sickness. A simple rule of thumb I often use is: *If the Lord made it, it's okay to eat.* So, cook and consume what God gave us.

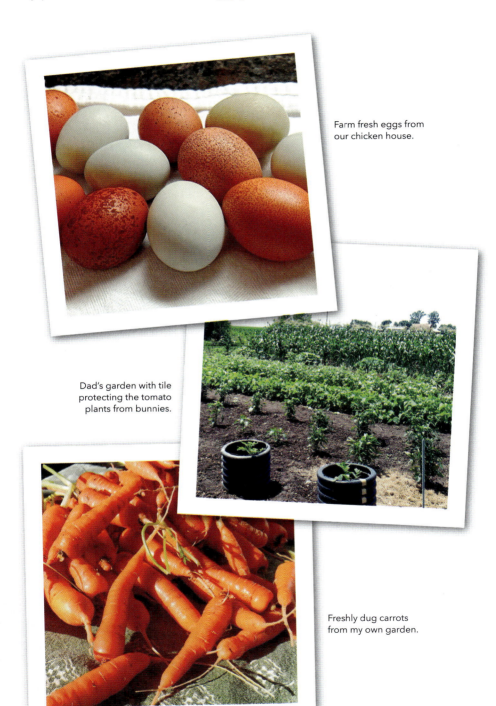

Farm fresh eggs from our chicken house.

Dad's garden with tile protecting the tomato plants from bunnies.

Freshly dug carrots from my own garden.

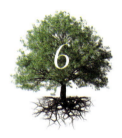

Zen in Motion:
Stress Management Techniques

Mom walks a mile and a half every single day. She always has ever since I can remember. It could be blizzarding, raining, hot and humid, or one of the windiest days on the planet, and she will get her walk in come hell or high water. Despite all the activities and chores that we did on our three acres, Mom always took a walk because she considered it quiet time, therapy.

One time in high school, I came home from the hairdresser's bawling my eyes out. The world seemed to be against me that day. I just got one of the worst perms ever—my long blonde hair turned completely frizzy from curls that were far too tight, even by early 1990s standards. I also had a growing cold sore on the right side of my mouth that seemed to be taking over my whole face. All I wanted to do was cry and hide. How could I go to school the next day looking so hideous?!

There was nothing Mom could do at that moment other than

suggest I call the hairdresser in the morning, schedule a follow-up hair appointment to try and fix the perm gone wrong, and to just get outside and take a walk. So, with tears flowing down my cheeks, I took Mom's advice and ventured down our gravel driveway onto the gravel road and walked the same route Mom walked every single day. By the time I finished the mile-and-a-half route, found some "smoothies" along the way to add to Mom's rock garden, and got back to the house, the tears had dried up, and my mindset had a more positive outlook. It wasn't the end of the world. The cold sore would eventually heal (hopefully overnight), and I could braid my hair until a better perm could be done.

Mom's walks on the long gravel roads by our acreage were more than just walks; they were the opportunity to get outdoors away from the confines of the house (and perhaps even her four children). Being outdoors and in nature is healing. There's nothing more enjoyable and stress-relieving than stepping outside for some fresh air and sunshine. Plus, regular walking has been shown to improve mood and overall mental well-being naturally, without the potential side effects of some medications.

And, if you're going to walk outdoors and enjoy nature, you might as well get a dog. We always had pets growing up; cats, dogs, rabbits, hamsters… Having a pet is proven to be therapy for reducing stress and anxiety. Pets give us unconditional love and friendship.

Get outdoors, go for a walk, enjoy nature, breathe in fresh air, absorb some sunshine, and take the dog. If you have a pet, they deserve exercise too.

Like walking, other forms of exercise prove to be effective in stress relief. Yoga is a great way to learn stress management. It teaches you to stay calm and composed, even in challenging poses—just as you would in stressful life situations—by maintaining steady breathing and a relaxed expression. Yoga is not only an excellent way to exercise, strengthen, and stretch your muscles but also a powerful practice for cultivating discipline and staying calm in difficult circumstances. The practice of yoga can be applied to life in general. The phrase, "Never let them see you sweat," perfectly captures this idea: staying cool, calm, and collected no matter the challenge.

Though I like yoga on occasion, my true sport is CrossFit. I have been doing it for well over a decade and love it for many reasons. Although it's different from yoga, it has taught me invaluable lessons over the years about facing challenges, overcoming fears, and navigating life's toughest trials. CrossFit has also helped me build the confidence to face new challenges head-on with a sense of clarity and calmness. Plus, it's incredibly effective at relieving stress. It has been my therapy over the years. It is my "me time."

Whatever your sport is, whatever you like to do for exercise, do it. There is no better stress relief than moving your body and accomplishing physical tasks, whether it is yoga, CrossFit, running, karate, swimming, biking, rucking…Exercise benefits not only our bodies but also our minds. By taking care of your body, you nourish your mind.

Our mental health is just as important as our physical health. Taking a moment to "breathe" and be mindful promotes mental clarity along with better heart health. It can also enhance relationships, training us to be aware of how our outward responses can affect those around us. Being mindful and taking a moment to reflect on our current situation is beneficial for us before we react to challenging situations, whether it is the demands of academics, your professional career, relationship struggles, financial worries, or any other stressful situation that life delivers you. It allows us to think more clearly and eliminate unnecessary stress and, sometimes, unconsciously projecting that stress onto those around us. Stress has a negative impact on our overall health. The impact of mental stress on heart health is significant, which only accelerates the aging process. And who wants to age faster? Being mindful takes practice and patience, but it's a powerful way to manage mental stress, reduce anxiety, and promote a healthy heart and stronger relationships.

When we are faced with challenging situations, our emotions can easily get away from us. It is crucial to hit the pause button and allow yourself a moment. Count to ten and take the time to consider your response (or reaction) thoughtfully. Visualize how your reaction may influence those around you and anticipate the potential consequences. Maintaining composure in tough circumstances not only earns you credibility and respect but also demonstrates maturity and poise. Remember, keeping a level head is far more effective than flying off the handle.

Keeping your composure also involves refraining from worrying about matters beyond your control. This is easier said than done but fixating on matters that you cannot change is a waste of energy and serves no purpose. The energy we spend worrying about things that cannot be changed, what has happened in the past, or what has not even happened yet in the future should be redirected to what is happening right now and in the present. Concentrate on what is within your control and free yourself of unnecessary worry that burns up your mental bandwidth.

Back in the day, you might have said that I was a bit of a drama queen (just a little) in my younger years. I loved the limelight and fed off attention, good, bad, and indifferent. I may have escalated stories when tattling on my sisters a few times or encouraged others around me to get involved in high school drama. But, like the story of the *Little Boy Who Cried Wolf*, over time, overexaggerating or blowing things out of proportion takes less effect. And sooner or later the people around you find you less reliable in your words and storytelling; trust starts to diminish. It is important to be genuine with your words and your actions. Avoid blowing things out of proportion.

Overreacting to trivial matters is not only unhealthy for your emotional well-being but also diminishes your credibility. Why amplify negativity when it's pointless and can be damaging? Stay grounded and refrain from overexaggerating situations. Be real. Be factual.

Like my younger years, there are people in the world who thrive off drama, even well into their adulthood. There is an addictive quality to drama that comes from the excitement and emotion one gets from it, yet at the same time, drama comes with a great deal of self-inflicted stress. Drama thrives on drama, and it fuels itself if you allow it to. The negative energy from drama is a total distraction that will easily suck you in, taking your focus away from where you should be. There's already too much negativity and drama in the world without adding more fuel to the fire. Drama creates conflict and can damage relationships, so avoid it at all costs.

Whether it is unnecessary drama or unfavorable situations that we find ourselves in, the way we reframe the situation can make a huge difference. We have the power to turn negativity into positivity by changing our perspectives. Finding the silver lining is important to help us change our outlook and the way we look at things. There are people I like to call "dark clouds" in the world: the negative Nellies, the naysayers. If possible, I try to avoid them. Nothing good ever comes from pessimism. Try to be optimistic wherever you go. Lift people up. Try to find the good in every situation. Be the light that enters the room, not the dark cloud.

Negative thinking not only impacts our mindset but inadvertently affects our appearance and the way we are perceived by others. Often, we're unaware that we may appear upset or unhappy, and our face and tone can overshadow what we are trying to say. So, make smiling a habit; not only does it make us appear more approachable, but it naturally corrects any negative tone in our voices. I've consistently reminded my children (especially if they come across as sarcastic) about "face and tone." When you are interacting with others, be aware of your own "face and tone." Our facial expressions and the tone of our voices can drastically change how we come across to others and alter the dynamics of any conversation. You've probably heard along the way that it takes more muscles to frown than it does to smile, so smile more!

Regardless of the challenges you may face, remind yourself that there's always a silver lining. Take stock of your blessings. List ten things you are grateful for before going to bed each night or keep a gratitude journal. Reminding yourself of the positives in your life will shift your perspective and foster a sense of gratitude versus a "woe is me" attitude.

People would much rather be around a ray of light than a dark cloud, and part of being that positive presence involves not taking things too personally—something I'm still working on myself. We might all be guilty of this because we care way too much about what other people think. Life won't come crashing down if someone is upset with you or if outcomes don't unfold as planned. It is not worth fretting about. Life continues regardless. The people you think might be upset at you for some reason might be having a bad day, or perhaps they are not aware of their "face and tone." Most people don't set out to be mean or intentionally hurt your feelings; and if they do, it's best not to give them a second thought. Why waste your energy on anyone who is purposely unkind and hurtful? Regardless, move on and invest your energy in people who care about you and the things that truly matter. How other people act and feel is out of our control, so cut yourself some slack and don't take what others say or do too personally. If you are treating people with honesty and kindness, you are doing your part.

Sometimes, doing our part requires selflessness, though it's debatable if true selflessness even exists. Many years ago, I had a deep conversation with a friend about the concept of being entirely selfless. He had asked me if there was anything in our human lives that we truly do without getting anything back in return. This was a very thought-provoking question, and we spent quite a bit of time thinking about it. We contemplated and discussed things we thought would qualify as 100% selfless, but none of them truly qualified as total selfless acts. We concluded that human beings get something out of anything we do, whether it is a response from another person or the feeling of contentment within ourselves. Ever since that very deep conversation, I think about giving selflessly often and try to give as selflessly as possible.

I encourage you to try and give as selflessly as possible without expecting anything in return. Whether it is a 'thank you,' an 'I love you,' or a gift, if you are expecting reciprocation, you are setting yourself up for disappointment when it does not happen. We should always do things for others because it comes from the heart, not for personal gain. Giving has been shown to trigger the release of oxytocin, a hormone that fosters feelings of warmth and connection. So, even when giving selflessly, you're still receiving the gift of positive emotions.

In recent years, I have really tried to explore ways to give better, to give with more meaning. Sending handwritten cards to those you care about for no reason (just because) and complimenting people you encounter (even strangers) are great ways to give without expecting anything in return. Calling up an old acquaintance just to check in to see how they have been doing or stopping by someone's house unexpectedly to drop off homemade cookies are other great ways to give that don't cost a lot of time or money.

Community work and volunteering are also awesome ways to give. In fact, research shows that people who volunteer have lower rates of depression, lower stress, and may live longer.[5] One of my favorite things to do over the years is picking up trash at parks, ball fields, and stadiums while I watch my kids participate in their sports activities. It's something that I have done that often goes unnoticed, but it makes me happy knowing that I've left the area much cleaner than how I found it. Though I've never sought recognition for picking up garbage, it's a small way for me to contribute positively to the community. If we all did more of these things, the world would be a better and more encouraging place to live.

We can all do a better job of dedicating our time and energy to activities that uplift us and foster positivity, while minimizing actions that contribute to negativity. We would all benefit from making an effort to eliminate distractions that have little or no impact on our lives—or, worse yet, a negative one. Personally, some practices that have significantly benefited me in recent years are silencing and turning all notifications off on my phone and reducing my intake of news on all platforms.

Remember those days of Saturday morning cartoons? Today, sadly, there are no more Saturday morning cartoons (unless you Google them on your iPhone or watch YouTube…and you can do that anytime, not just on Saturday mornings). News programming fills not only Saturday mornings but Sunday mornings too. News programming takes up almost every hour of every single day. There is absolutely no break from it. The news is hard to avoid, with notifications and headlines bombarding us everywhere, whether it is on television, streaming on our mobile phones, or checking the heaps of news apps available on our devices. AND…back in the days of Saturday morning cartoons, your television stations signed off at midnight, giving viewers a forced break from too much TV time.

Here are some descriptive words from just the first segment of a national morning newscast that I watched recently: deadly, outbreak, massive destruction, violent, threat, dangerous, damaging, rough, battle, restrictions, delays, allegations, mishandled, unstable, killing, collapse, violations, fatal, defects, hazardous, neglected, demolition, mayhem, injury, wrongdoing, warnings, urgent. If there were any positive words at all, they were completely smothered by these negative words.

And we wonder why depression and suicide rates are at all-time highs. If it bleeds, it leads. Good news doesn't sell. We are all consuming too much news, and it is affecting our overall well-being.

We do not need all the rings, dings, and distractive bubbles popping up every ten seconds. Even without the sounds, for some of us visually seeing those little red bubbles are cues to pick up our phone and respond immediately. They give us permission to look at our phone to answer email and text messages, see how many "likes" we've received, respond to Snapchat, know what news just broke, or what our current weather situation looks like. It is exhausting and it is stressful.

Though news can be negative and draining, so can social media. Limit your time on social media. Even if your notifications are turned off, stop checking for the "likes" and responses to your posts. Social media is a dark and deep rabbit hole that can negatively impact your well-being along with being a giant time suck. Know that everyone's stories are their highlight reels. Social media is not real life. The average person spends over two hours on social media and scrolls through 300 feet of mobile content every day! Read a book, go for a walk, or create a homemade meal instead!

Think of the hundreds of things we could enjoy so much more if our noses were not in our phones all the time. Put the phone up, turn the television off, and listen to music instead. Music can be extremely helpful in reducing stress and anxiety by reducing our cortisol levels—the stress hormone. When I was a teenager, I would spend hours in my bedroom just listening to music. Music has always had a positive impact on my mood. The power of lyrics to influence the mind is truly remarkable. Music serves as a means of escape and can cultivate a more optimistic outlook on life. Today, I still listen to music, whether it is in the car alone, singing at the top of my lungs, or while I am at home doing chores around the house. Turning off the TV and listening to music can provide a break from visual stimulation and offer a chance to focus on auditory experiences. It helps us relax and sparks creativity and emotional expression.

It's also refreshing to completely disconnect from all electronics and simply enjoy dinner around the table. Use mealtime as a time to connect with others and have meaningful conversations. Savor mealtime as a celebration of nutrition and nourishment for the body. Rather than eating at your desk or in front of the TV in your living room, create dedicated spaces for meals to avoid mindless eating. Taking the time to enjoy good food with good people with no distractions is a lost art.

> 66 *Eating without conversation is only stoking.*
> —Marcelene Cox, American writer

It saddens me to learn that only 30% of American families eat together at the family table nowadays. Sharing a meal and discussing the events of the day is about much more than simply consuming food together. Family dinners can prevent issues with eating disorders, alcohol and substance abuse, violent behavior, depression, and suicidal thoughts in adolescents. Make each meal a mindful experience that you can fully enjoy by eating slowly and savoring every bite. Recognize the significance of food in our lives and enjoy the company with whom we share our meals.

Fruity Shrimp Stir-Fry

2 tablespoons unrefined Extra-Virgin Olive Oil
2 minced Garlic Cloves
1 cup Celery (sliced)
1 cup small Broccoli Florets
1 cup fresh Mushrooms (sliced)
1 lb. fresh rinsed Shrimp
1 cup Pineapple (cubed)
2 Peaches (cubed)
4 Green Onions (chopped)
½ cup fresh Cilantro (optional)
1 tablespoon Red Pepper Flakes
4 cups of Jasmine Rice

To start this family favorite, put the olive oil in a large pan or skillet. Heat and add the minced garlic. Brown the garlic and add the chopped vegetables. Sauté the vegetables until the broccoli turns dark green and becomes slightly tender. Add the fresh shrimp. Once the shrimp starts to turn white, add the fruit, cilantro, red pepper flakes, and sea salt. Stir and serve over rice. Serves 4.

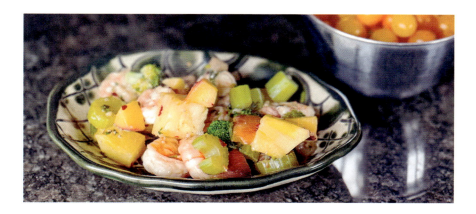

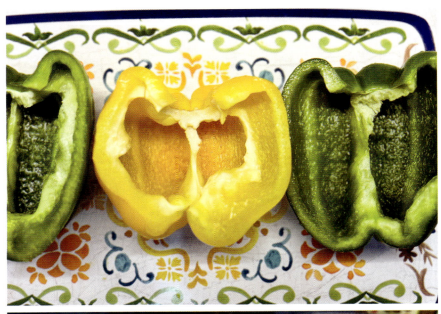
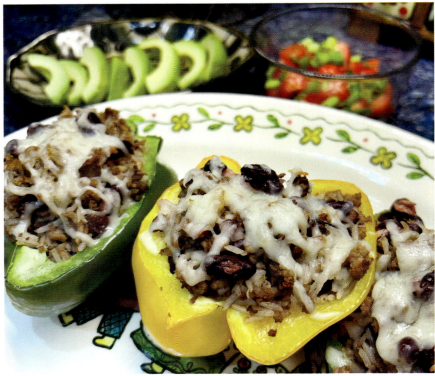

Amazing Stuffed Peppers

3 Bell Peppers (cut in half top to bottom/symmetrical)
2 lbs. Ground Turkey
1 can Red Kidney Beans
1-1/2 cups Cooked Rice
1 diced Jalapeño
3 diced Green Onions
1/2 diced Purple Onion
1 teaspoon Cajun Pepper
1 teaspoon Garlic Powder
1 teaspoon Cumin
Shredded Cheddar Cheese

Brown the ground turkey in a pan. Drain and rinse the kidney beans. Add the kidney beans and the rice to the ground turkey. Add the diced onions and jalapeños along with the spices. Cook on low for a few minutes to get the flavors hopping.

Spoon and stuff the ground turkey mix into the halved peppers and place in a cake pan. You will likely have leftover turkey mix that can be used as leftovers for taco salads, burritos, or a healthier nacho. Top each stuffed pepper with shredded cheddar cheese. Pour 1/3 cup water into the bottom of the cake pan (or cookie sheet) so the peppers can steam and soften while in the oven. Bake at 350°F for 30-40 minutes. Serve hot with fresh guacamole, pico de gallo, and tortilla chips.

Like sharing a spectacular meal with friends or family, focus on experiences rather than material things. Experiences create lasting memories and enrich our lives in ways that possessions simply cannot. When our two children were little, they would get theater or concert tickets, registration to a camp that they wanted to participate in, or a fun family vacation for Christmas and birthdays instead of a lot of toys. These great gifts gave them experiences that they loved and fewer "things" to clutter the house. When we bought "things" for our kids as gifts, we chose items that encouraged learning and fun activities, such as books, LEGOs®, puzzles, and sports equipment. Many times, these "things" were all shared as a family and made for wonderful memories. My rule for learning materials is the same as my rule for fruit and vegetables—unlimited. I always told my kids that if I could afford it, they could have as many books and puzzles as they wanted.

Feeding the mind is just as important as feeding the body, but just like our minds, our homes can become cluttered—full of things that take up unnecessary space. While it's natural to be emotionally attached to certain things in our lives, whether it is our grandmother's recipe box, a figurine we got while on vacation, or a sportscar in the garage, detaching our emotions from "things" can contribute to a more balanced and fulfilling life and allows us to adapt more easily to changes in our lives. My husband and I just experienced this ourselves as we downsized from our five-bedroom home to a two-bedroom condo. The number of "things" we had accumulated over the years was astronomical, and deciding what stayed and what went was a tough job. We had to get rid of a lot of "things" with memories attached to them. But at the end of the move, it felt good to downsize. We have what we need to live comfortably, and life seems a bit easier too, without all the stuff. Though we have let go of many "things" we were emotionally attached to, we still cherish years of wonderful memories of living in that five-bedroom house with our two kids.

Emotional detachment from material things grants you a sense of freedom, inner peace, and enlightenment. Decluttering our minds and the spaces where we live can both be very therapeutic. Getting rid of stuff that just sits around and clutters our lives is freeing. Most of the time, we are attached to "things" because we have memories attached to them. Let go and remember that the memories attached to your "things" are far more meaningful than the objects themselves. Memories stay with us forever, without ever accumulating dust.

By embracing simplicity and appreciating life's essentials, we can focus on what truly matters, rather than succumbing to the pressure of trying to "keep up with the Joneses." It is like we are all in a contest or race with one another as to who has the biggest and best of everything. We all want big, beautiful houses, newer cars, and designer clothing, but all these luxuries can bring complexity. Ultimately, when our time on Earth comes to an end, we cannot take money or material goods with us. Instead, focus on life's simple pleasures. The simple things often hold a much greater value than the complexities we burden ourselves with in the chase to have the biggest and the best. The difference between wants and needs lies in self-control, and there's a deep sense of peace that comes from mastering it.

More than material things, the individuals we surround ourselves with undoubtedly influence our lives in some incredible ways. Sometimes, we need to declutter the people we surround ourselves with. Choose to surround yourself with people who respect you and lift you up. It's important to recognize that there are individuals in the world who thrive on drama and negativity, seeking to bring others down. We may have family members or friends who are "dark clouds" in our lives. Be mindful of these individuals, realize how they impact our well-being, and have ways to mitigate their negative influence on us.

No matter who and what we surround ourselves with, remember to always prioritize yourself; you are your own greatest asset. By taking care of your own needs first, you strengthen your ability to support and be there for those who rely on you. Developing a healthy mental state not only benefits you in many ways, but it also positively influences those around you.

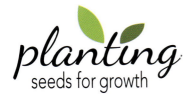

Reminders for Self-Care

- Be patient and compassionate with yourself and treat yourself with the same kindness and understanding you would offer to a friend.

- Set realistic, achievable goals for personal growth, and look forward to the possibilities your future holds.

- Find satisfaction with who you are in the present moment, and nurture self-love as a foundation for personal well-being.

- Recognize your unique strengths, talents, and positive qualities. Take time to celebrate your achievements, big or small.

- Create healthy boundaries to safeguard your well-being and prioritize what truly matters. Every commitment is a choice, so focus your energy wisely.

- Focus on what aligns with your goals and values.

- Take time to rest and recharge. Prioritize sleep and relaxation.

- Engage in activities that bring you joy and replenish your spirit, whether it's a hobby, a walk in nature, or quality time with loved ones.

- Practice gratitude daily by reflecting on the positive aspects of your life and those around you.

The world can be complex, and the burdens we carry—whether they involve material goods or the people we surround ourselves with—can feel heavy. Stress is an inevitable part of life, touching each of us daily, adding to the challenges we face. Chronic stress can have significant health implications. Managing stress is challenging, especially given the current high rates of mental illness and depression. Know that seeking professional help is not only acceptable but also commendable. There are times when we require more support than we can manage alone, and it's important—for both us and those we care about—to reach out for assistance.

I have personally sought the guidance of a counselor during periods when I faced challenges both personally and professionally. These were moments when I truly needed someone to help me navigate through complex emotions and thoughts, which could have otherwise been extremely detrimental. Sometimes, merely having someone to talk to can make a significant difference, while at other times, the issues may run much deeper. It's concerning that over half of individuals wrestling with mental illness choose not to seek treatment.[6] We need to change this statistic and encourage mental health counseling to help us strengthen our overall well-being. It is okay to not be okay.

❝ *Stress acts as an accelerator: it will push you either forward or backward, but you choose which direction.*
—Chelsea Erieau, Writer and Sociologist

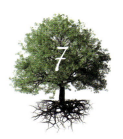

Recharge & Renew:
Rest and Relaxation Strategies

In the pea-picking days, our family had a black and white TV that only got two channels: CBS and PBS. On very special occasions like birthdays or slumber parties, Mom would rent a VCR from the video store in Algona, Iowa, along with movies on VCR tape. Remember the days of "be kind and rewind"? It was much different than the movies we get on-demand today. During a regular week, my sisters and I would watch maybe two to three hours of TV a day (if we were lucky) *Little House on the Prairie* after school and one hour or so of TV at night before bedtime, sitcoms primarily. On weekends, we loved watching Bob Ross (the artist) and Julia Childs (the chef) on Iowa Public Television. Both public television celebrities left us inspired to create beautiful paintings and amazing culinary dishes (or at least try to) during the weekends when we couldn't get outside due to unfavorable Iowa weather. But *Dukes of Hazard* was our favorite program of all time and was on Friday nights. Friday nights were the best with Bo and Luke Duke. After our family ate supper (I call it dinner today), we all looked forward to the one or two hours of primetime television that we would watch together. Bedtime was routinely at 8:00 or 8:30 for all of us, except for Mom and Dad, who would maybe stay up an extra hour or so.

Limited television and a routine bedtime were unspoken rules at our house growing up. We never whined about going to bed early or begged to stay up any later to watch the next television program. A good night's sleep was important because we all had busy days ahead of us, even on most weekends. Routine was important then and still is today. We all need an adequate amount of sleep; 6-8 hours a night, in fact. Going without enough sleep does not just make you tired; it also contributes to chronic health problems, including heart disease, obesity, type 2 diabetes, and depression. Sleep affects our memory, cognitive performance, emotional regulation, and our creative thinking. And sleep can strengthen the lymphatic system, which strengthens the immune system. Getting sufficient sleep, along with the good nutrition that Mom and Dad provided us, is undoubtedly why we rarely had any "sick days" from school. We all were as healthy as a horse growing up which has transitioned well into our later years.

For the most part, we went to bed when it was dark and got up with the sun. In the summertime, we were allowed to stay up a little later naturally, with longer days and no school. The days of routine bedtime in many households are a thing of the past. Children today are not only overfed and malnourished from eating a diet mostly of processed foods and sugars, but they are sleep-deprived.

Twenty percent of American children use melatonin for sleep.[7] Our country has seen a rapid rise in pediatric melatonin use due to sleep problems attributed to an increase in mental illness and screen use.

Like the routine I had growing up, my two children went to bed at 8:30 every night, especially on school nights. Phones and TVs were not allowed in bedrooms either. Technology is too much of a temptation that keeps you from much-needed rest. They never argued about it, though both kids would casually bring up that their friends got to stay up later at night and their friends got to use their cell phones to play video games and watch videos in their bedrooms. But it was never a fight. The rules we set for both kids were just how it was, and both of our children accepted them; it was routine, and it was our schedule.

Thanks to the good sleeping habits instilled in my sisters and me when we were young, I rarely rely on an alarm to wake up in the morning; I naturally am up and ready to start my day once the sun starts to peek through the windows. Perhaps it's due to the lifelong routine I've maintained, but I prefer to believe it's my attunement to the circadian rhythm. Sunrise and sunset naturally influence our circadian rhythms. It's the way nature intended it to be. Humans are meant to sleep at night and be up and active and eat during the day.

When we are active during the day we are naturally ready for rest at night; our bodies need it. Reducing time spent with technology by at least an hour before bed helps with a better night's sleep too. And cool temperatures are also recommended to sleep well. As your body cools, melatonin is naturally released by the pineal gland in the brain; no supplement needed. A healthy diet can also provide us with melatonin. Pistachios, tart cherries, kiwis, fatty fish, eggs, and milk are great foods that are high in melatonin. So, there is a reason a warm glass of milk before bed can help us sleep better.

What we eat, how much we eat, and when we eat can also impact how well we sleep. Avoid big meals right before bedtime for better digestion and improved sleep. We should eat during the daylight (when the sun is up). Start your day with a healthy breakfast, make lunch your largest meal, and follow it with a lighter dinner (or supper). Aim for a 14-16 hour intermittent fast to support your overall health.

Your body needs a break from eating and time to recharge. Our bodies were not meant to snack all day and all night long. Nighttime is for rest, a time for our bodies to rebuild and restore, not for snacking.

When we sleep well, we should be ready to get up with the sun. Enjoying the sunrise is a wonderful way to start your day. Experience the beauty of both the sunrise and sunset. Taking the time to appreciate nature and admire the power of the sun is good for our mental health and a wonderful relaxation strategy. This is why so many people love to watch the sunset when they are on vacation. Have you ever been on vacation, and groups of people literally just stop what they are doing and take the time to watch the sun slowly go down over the horizon? There is something about the sun that is magical, giving us renewed energy and appreciation for life. It never gets old, with every sunrise and sunset producing a variety of stunning colors and different patterns throughout the endless sky.

Watching the sunset is often an appreciated part of a vacation, symbolizing rest and relaxation—so why not bring a little of that vacation mindset into your daily life and routine? Of course, nothing compares to the rejuvenation and inspiration that come from stepping away completely—so make it a priority to plan regular vacations that allow you to truly disconnect and recharge. If I had unlimited funds, I would travel the world. Unfortunately, vacationing full-time is not practical. Vacations cost money, and if you have the means, travel more. There are magnificent sights to see in the world (near and far) that will simply take your breath away. Everyone should see the mountains, swim in the ocean, and visit a foreign country. Having lived in Iowa all my life, I find mountains and oceans mysterious since, for most of my life, I was surrounded by cornfields. Whatever your ideal vacation spot might be—whether it's a far-off destination or the iconic Field of Dreams in Iowa—make it a point to take time off and explore the world around you for a variety of beneficial reasons.

The first real vacation I ever went on was to the Black Hills. I was fourteen, and at the time, Mom and Dad had a long white Dodge Aspen station wagon with brown wood trim. It was a luxury vehicle back then. All six of us could fit comfortably in it, and so we drove that station wagon eight hours from Fenton, Iowa, to the Black Hills in South Dakota. I remember riding in the very back so I could lay down and listen to my Walkman cassette player while seeing how many different state license plates we could spot along the interstate. All four of us girls fought as to who got to ride in the back and Mom and Dad made us take turns throughout the drive.

Our trip to the Black Hills resembled scenes from the movie *National Lampoon's Family Vacation*, starring Chevy Chase. Dad loved that movie. That was one of the very few "real" vacations we took growing up. Vacations were few and far between, probably due to family finances and Mom and Dad having to take time off work. Our family, however, often took weekend getaways, packing a cooler full of bologna sandwiches and driving two or three hours to amusement parks like Valleyfair in Shakopee, Minnesota, or Adventureland in Des Moines, Iowa. We also spent time at nearby lakes, enjoying fishing trips and outdoor picnics filled with simple, wholesome fun.

❝ *We are always getting ready to live, but never living.*
—Ralph Wa do Emerson, American Poet

When I was at the height of my career; I cannot remember one year where I used all my paid vacation time. According to a 2023 Pew Research Center survey, 48% of workers in the United States don't use all their vacation days.[8] Americans are terrible at using vacation time because we are worried that we will fall behind, think it could cost us our job, keep us from getting promoted, and/or we feel bad about our workload falling on others. My advice to you is to use ALL your paid vacation time. It is YOUR time. It is time that you have earned. Vacation time, whether you spend it in the mountains, the ocean, or in your backyard, is valuable. Vacation is your time to recharge your batteries and unplug. We all require a recharge, or we become completely depleted.

Be mindful and be intentional about getting YOU time. If you do not take care of yourself, you will become less effective in fulfilling the needs of those who rely on you. I will remind you that it is not selfish to take care of you first, ever. Read a book, get a massage, go for a long walk or go to the gym, get a manicure or pedicure, listen to music, have coffee with a friend, or just appreciate quiet time alone. Quiet time alone gives us all much-needed time to think, organize our thoughts, and even be creative. We all need a mental and physical break from the daily grind.

When we were kids there were moments of silence when we would just lay in the grass and look up at the sky. It was so peaceful, and it felt so good to have the soft, cool grass underneath us and to breathe in the smells of the countryside. We would do this in the wintertime too, fully dressed in snowsuits with our hoods up over our heads and knitted mittens on our hands. We would just lay there in the quiet cold, and for some reason, it just felt good. No noise. No homework or chores. No playing or fighting—just stillness.

Sufficient rest and relaxation serve as effective stress management techniques. When we're exhausted, we are not our best selves. So, it's crucial to slow down, take breaks, prioritize rest, and get enough sleep.

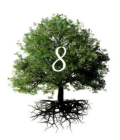

Conquering Healthy Challenges:
Personal Growth & Thriving

    From the time I was old enough to get a job, I had one. Before I had my driver's license, I would babysit neighbor kids and work in the fields for local farmers. I wanted to make money for two reasons: so I could buy the occasional outfit at Brass Buckle, and so I could save up to afford a college education after high school. Early on, I knew that a degree was in my future. Both of my grandfathers and my dad went into the military and Mom went to college but never graduated. I wanted to go to college and graduate with a degree from a college or university. It was important to me. To get that degree meant I would need money to pay for that higher education that I so desperately wanted.

    The toughest job I ever had during those early working years was field work. This included picking up rocks, walking or riding beans, and detasseling corn. When you look across a farm field and it is hundreds of acres in size; doing any of these jobs is a challenge. To put it into perspective, there are 640 acres in one square mile. And

CONQUERING HEALTHY CHALLENGES

99

most square miles around Fenton, Iowa, were filled with nothing but soybean and corn fields.

- Picking up rocks always took place in the spring, before crops were planted. The farmer would drive up and down the empty field rows, and workers would either ride on or walk alongside the moving hayrack being pulled by the tractor, spot large rocks that could get caught in planting or harvesting equipment, pick up the rock, and throw it on the hayrack. Then the worker would either jump back on the hayrack or walk beside the hayrack depending on how "rocky" the terrain was. When the hayrack was full of rocks or the workday was done, the rocks collected on the hayrack would generally be dumped in one big pile somewhere on the farmer's property or in a ditch alongside one of his fields.

- Walking beans consisted of walking up and down rows of soybeans with either an old-fashioned garden hoe or a handheld spray bottle of Round-up to eliminate weeds. Riding beans was much easier because it used the modern technology of what looked like a long beam that was attached to the front of a tractor. Along this beam were four seats mounted facing forward: two on each side of the tractor. Riders would have giant wands that were hooked up to a large tank of weed killer attached to the tractor and riders would spray the weeds that would come up through the rows of soybeans or corn.

- Detasseling corn involved walking rows upon rows of corn and pulling the tassels off the tops of each corn plant. The purpose of detasseling corn is to prevent unwanted pollination, ensuring the production of pure hybrid seed corn. Detasseling corn was the worst of all fieldwork because it typically took place in mid-July to early-August when the corn was tall enough to have grown tassels (about shoulder height) and the Iowa summer weather was at its hottest. You also had to wear boots, jeans, and long-sleeved shirts to avoid getting cut by corn leaves. Imagine hundreds of paper cuts all over your legs and arms while sweating to death.

Regardless of the task at hand, standing before an endless field prompts two immediate questions: "Where do we even start?" and "How long will it take?" Like the ten gallons of peas that needed shucking, beginning field work seemed like an insurmountable task. But one rock at a time, one weed at a time, or one corn tassel at a time, it all miraculously got done. It might have taken days or even weeks, but it all got done. A challenge in the beginning turned into a huge accomplishment in the end. A job well done and a paycheck collected. Both were accomplishments to be proud of.

Continuously challenge yourself by seeking out tasks, projects, hobbies, and adventures that push you beyond your comfort zone. Get comfortable with the uncomfortable. Embracing discomfort fosters confidence and mental resilience. While venturing outside your comfort zone may seem scary, it opens doors to new opportunities and growth.

Saving money for college was a challenge that introduced me to additional hurdles along the way, like field work. I had the goal of graduating from college, and to get there, I had to face many obstacles. At a young age, I was ready for some of those encounters and not-so-ready for others. Looking back, I see how important it is to approach each challenge with a sense of purpose and adaptability. To prepare yourself as best as possible for any challenge, establish clear goals and look to the journey ahead. Know that the road might be difficult at times, but it will be worth it. Take the time to write your goals down and create a plan to accomplish them. Don't be afraid to dream big. Create a bucket list and post it on your refrigerator or keep it inside your journal. Having goals provides motivation and opportunities for personal growth. Challenge yourself, remain curious, and seek out new and exciting goals to pursue once you've achieved your current ones. Having goals is a healthy part of life, providing direction and motivation to move forward with purpose and focus.

To help me plan my dream of going to college, I remember having a meeting with our high school guidance counselor during my senior year of high school. He recommended a few two-year business schools and community colleges and then proceeded to tell me, "The only degree you will be getting is your M-R-S degree." I'm not sure if he was dead serious or sarcastic, but either way, his words would not fly in today's world, and they really pissed me off back then. In fact, his inappropriate words gave me the fuel to prove him wrong. Not only did I get an Associate of Arts degree in Business, but I received a Bachelor of Arts degree as well. Later in my career, after starting a family and getting my M-R-S degree, I pursued my Master of Science degree in Psychology as I continued to set new goals for myself, aiming to become one of the youngest women in management at a renowned media company. I accomplished both my academic and career goals during the completion of my thesis. Check and CHECK!

Accomplish something every single day. It does not have to be something big like a college degree or getting a promotion. It can be something as simple as just making your bed. Avoid what I call "zero days." Zero days are days when you accomplish absolutely nothing. Keep in mind that rest days do not count as "zero days." During rest days, you are accomplishing a much-needed recharge. Even on rest days, you can accomplish something small like rewriting your to-do list, reading an interesting article, ordering the next book you want to read, or watching an educational documentary.

Just as accomplishing small daily tasks builds a sense of progress and purpose, participating in sports can foster discipline, perseverance, and teamwork—qualities that translate into everyday life. Whether you're tackling a personal to-do list or working toward athletic goals, the effort you put in matters.

And when it comes to showcasing effort, sports provide an incredible stage to demonstrate dedication and perseverance. I am a firm believer in participating in athletics for so many reasons. Sports can offer countless opportunities for growth and achievement, whether through individual interests or as part of a team. Being on a team can teach invaluable lessons, even if you're not the star player. Maybe you're on the "B" team, an alternate, or have a challenging coach or teammate. Regardless, your role is essential. Supporting teammates, offering advice, sharpening your skills, or leading by example in practices all contribute to the team's success. Beyond improving your abilities, being part of a team instills patience, grit, and the understanding that every contribution, big or small, has value.

Compared to team sports, individual sports offer a different set of challenges and can be just as beneficial. It is just you (all you and no one else) against other competitive individuals. I participated in track in high school, not because I was good at it, but because it kept me in shape. I was not fast but did have decent endurance and was strong for my size. So, my preferred events were the shot put and the 2-mile run. I got a kick out of being the smallest girl who showed up at the shot put circle to check in and have fellow shot-putters look at me like it was a joke. There was a certain confidence that was built in doing the shot put just by showing up and having people doubt your abilities. I never won, but I placed third a few times and could hold my own. The 3,200-meter race was both physically and mentally challenging. Eight laps around the track seemed like an eternity. I detested it but did it anyway because I knew it would make me a better athlete overall and it was the first event after the field events, so I could have both my events completed before most of the other runners even started. It was nice to be done, somewhat relax, enjoy some snacks, and cheer on my teammates during the rest of the track meet.

Many times, we can get discouraged because we focus our attention on others and their accomplishments (i.e., the athlete who threw the shot put farthest or the one next to you in the 3,200-meter run). And, though it is nice to win, it is also an amazing feeling to have beaten your own distance or time, setting a new personal record. When we concentrate on how others perform, we can be intimidated, and our heads then fill with self-doubt and insecurities. Negative thoughts such as "I could never do that," "I don't have time," "maybe this isn't for me," "maybe tomorrow," or "maybe next year" are simply forms of self-sabotage or excuses that prevent us from taking action. And excuses only hold you back and prevent you from moving forward. Know that you are capable of more than you think. Viewing others' accomplishments with intimidation is the wrong perspective to take when facing your own challenges. Instead, let their achievements inspire and motivate you to reach your potential. Remember, challenges are an opportunity to push yourself, not to compete with others.

"The only way to eat an elephant is one bite at a time" is a saying we hear often, and it is so true. Like picking up rocks in a large Iowa field, it is one rock at a time to get the job done. If it is getting a college degree, it might be completing one class at a time. If you want to run a marathon, it starts with one step forward to build momentum. Focus on that momentum and simply move forward one step (or one bite) at a time. Celebrate the small wins. Be your own cheerleader. And follow your plan.

I am not doing any field work these days or running track, but I have been doing CrossFit since 2012 and every day is not any less challenging. I have done thousands of CrossFit workouts; every single one has been intimidating as hell. Strength and endurance are not the only things that have been enhanced, but I have learned new athletic skills, how to keep my composure in stressful situations, and have developed resilience and an even stronger self-confidence. I know how to breathe, to pace myself; not to shoot out of the gate too quickly despite what the athlete next to me does. I've learned to be more mindful and aware of my capabilities both in the gym and in everyday life.

CrossFit competitions are even more mentally demanding (and I've participated in a few). Competing in front of an audience can amplify nerves and self-doubt, but there's no time to dwell on failure—you must move forward. Focus on the moment, be present, have fun, and know that in the end, you will have done your very best. CrossFit workouts provide me with physical and mental challenges, and the sport itself has taught me how to thrive in everyday situations. The CrossFit community is a group of wonderful, like-minded individuals who have all been uplifting and supportive, which has been a huge bonus. Very rarely will you find a Cross-Fitter who is negative and not willing to help a fellow athlete.

When I started CrossFit, I couldn't do a 10-inch box jump, and I was far from completing even one pull-up. Along the way, there have been failures (no reps), uncompleted workouts (due to time caps), and plenty of frustrations, but I stuck with it and continued to challenge myself. CrossFit, like any sport, requires hard work and dedication to improve. Today, I can do 24-inch box jumps and string together several pull-ups with ease. I've also learned to do pistols (one-legged squats) and can effortlessly perform handstand push-ups. These achievements didn't happen overnight—it took hundreds of classes and workouts to get here. The sense of accomplishment I've gained in this sport has been worth every challenging workout over the years, but success has come one movement at a time, one workout at a time, and one day at a time through consistent practice and determination.

Over the years, I've sought out and embraced many other challenges that have prompted personal growth, boosted my self-confidence, and introduced me to some truly remarkable individuals. Here are a few suggestions that I hope will inspire your own journey of personal growth:

- Travel (take a trip).
- Visit a new church.
- Drop in as a visitor to a gym in a new city.
- Sign up for a cooking class.
- Get dressed up and eat at a nice restaurant.
- Sing karaoke.
- Play a musical instrument.
- Do a workout at a public park with a group of friends.
- Try a new sport like pickleball, rock-climbing, or CrossFit.
- Apply for your dream job.
- Adopt a pet.
- Take dance lessons.
- Sign up for a simple 3k run or something as big as a triathlon.
- Strike up a conversation with a stranger.
- Write poetry or start writing your own book.
- Learn to use chopsticks.
- Go fishing and bait your own hook.
- Paint a picture or an entire room in your house.
- Hike in a national park.
- Learn and play a new card game.
- Go for a swim in a lake or the ocean.
- Learn to scuba dive.
- Study a foreign language.
- Step into the saddle and go horseback riding.

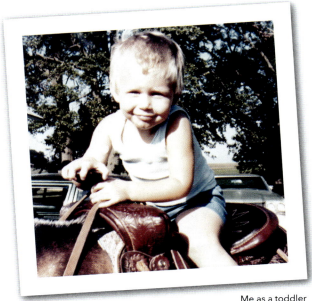

Me as a toddler
sitting on our horse, Chief.

I encourage you to find new challenges, whatever they might be. Test yourself. Adapt to new environments and learn new skills. Move outside of your comfort zone. Know that you are capable of anything you put your mind to. Start today. Start now. Stay at it. You will thank yourself tomorrow…and most definitely will thank yourself ten years from now.

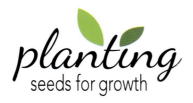 9 Benefits of Challenging Yourself

---

1. Builds confidence
2. Teaches you through mistakes and failures
3. Keeps you humble
4. Sharpens your focus
5. Reduces the fear of bigger challenges
6. Enhances problem solving skills
7. Produces newfound energy and drive
8. Creates a sense of accomplishment
9. Nurtures overall life success

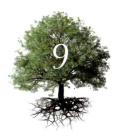

Dollars & Sense:
Financial Fitness

    Mom would shop at used clothing stores to keep her four girls in the latest fashions, with The Mercantile in Fenton being one of her go-to spots. And, when we were not wearing consignment clothes, we were wearing hand-me-downs. I was lucky to be the oldest. The summer going into my freshman year of high school, I really wanted designer jeans from Brass Buckle— desperately. I remember shopping with my mom at The Mercantile in Fenton and finding a pair of *Pepe* jeans, which were the style back then, along with *Z Cavaricci* and *Guess*. The *Pepe* jeans I found fit perfectly and were like a brand-new pair of jeans to me. From Brass Buckle, they would have cost at least $75, but we got them for $3 used and barely worn. I remember going to school wearing my "brand new" pair of *Pepe* jeans and feeling so proud and so cool. All I wanted to do was to fit in and be noticed. But it did not take long for that feeling to deflate when a few upper-class girls walked by with one very popular girl announcing to her group and in front of everyone else in the school hallway, "Oh my gosh, those are my old jeans she has on. My mom took them to the used clothing store last month." The group of girls giggled and walked off. I was definitely noticed, all right, and I had never been so embarrassed in my entire teenage life.

Thrifting was very common when we were growing up. Mom did not think anything of it. But back in my preteen and teen years, I was really embarrassed by it. Sometimes, I even sat in the car with the seat laid back so no one would see me at a used clothing store while Mom went in to do her shopping. However, it was a way for our family to save money and still provide us with what we needed and even sometimes what we really wanted, like a pair of *Pepe* or *Guess* jeans. As I have gotten older and understand the value of the dollar, shopping at consignment stores has been a great way for my own family to save money now too. I even brag to others about how little I spend on secondhand designer finds.

During high school, I worked multiple jobs to save money for college and for a few clothing items that I chose to buy brand new, which was a luxury. Like many preteen girls, I started out babysitting for one dollar an hour per child. To put $1/hour into perspective, gas was under one dollar per gallon at the time. There were a few families within a ten-mile radius who would hire me occasionally on the weekends. During the two summers that I was 13 and 14 years old, I babysat for a farming family who had two little girls. This was a good, consistent summer gig, Monday through Friday from 8:00 a.m. until 5:00 p.m. They paid me $5 an hour and it was decent money for summer work. $5 an hour was good, but walking beans and picking up field rocks made even better money at $10 or more an hour. Those jobs were much harder and taxing on the body than watching two little girls, and the hours were longer, usually starting promptly at sun-up.

Once I got a driver's license I could get a real job, which I did right away. Being a waitress at the Algona Pizza Hut was fun. It was not a lot of money, but when the cooks in the kitchen made mistakes on pizzas, I would get the chance to take these mistakes home for the rest of the family to enjoy. Sometimes, call-ins did not come in to pick up their pizza, so they would have to be thrown out for safety reasons (just like the cooks' mistake pizzas), which I never understood. So, I would volunteer to take them to the dumpster, setting them safely aside so I could rescue them after my shift. Needless to say, Mom, Dad, and my sisters ate a lot of pizza during that time, and I remember how good it felt to "provide" for my family.

The local truck stop in Algona, Iowa, consisted of a gas station and a diner known for serving hearty breakfast and delicious pie. The diner, the Chrome Country Inn, was my next waitressing stint, which was an upgrade from Pizza Hut. Waitressing was fun, and the tips were better than at Pizza Hut, so I worked every Saturday and Sunday morning starting between 5:00 and 6:00 a.m. and worked until midafternoon my sophomore through senior years in high school. During those same years I was also a lifeguard during the summers at the Burt Community Pool, which was twelve miles east of Fenton and ten miles north of Algona. Having multiple jobs at one time was normal and pretty common. Most kids my age were eager to make money.

Once I got into college, the City of Burt promoted me to the manager of the Burt Community Pool, along with lifeguarding in the afternoons, which came with a nice raise. They also hired me in the mornings as their local garbage gal (yes, I rode on the back of the garbage truck, tossing garbage cans full of stinky garbage into the back of a huge, smelly garbage truck). Like Dad, I loved the challenge of a good workout, and slinging garbage kept me in great shape. So, on my summer mornings during the week, I worked for the city picking up garbage, painting Burt City Hall, and doing other odd jobs around the tiny town of Burt, Iowa. In the afternoons, I managed the operations of the town's community pool, taught swimming lessons, and lifeguarded. And I still worked at the Chrome Country Inn on weekends when I could.

My early work experience is a prime example of becoming financially fit. For those less fortunate who don't have money handed to them, getting a job to pay for the things you need and to save for the things you want is necessary. Mom and Dad taught us an incredible work ethic, and that has been passed down to my two children, who have also worked multiple jobs starting in their teen years to afford the things important to them, including their college educations.

Once you start to make money, knowing what to do with it is another matter. My first full-time job after graduating with a two-year associate's degree in business was with a financial planning firm. While employed at Agnew Young & Associates (I was the associate), I learned the importance of investing. My job as an executive assistant was to create the investment summaries for the firm's clients when they came in for financial planning meetings (aka financial checkups). These financial summaries illustrated how each client's investments were performing over time and helped them plan and prepare for their financial goals. I witnessed clients who would rollover their employer's 401(k)s into mutual funds or annuities with the firm. I also saw how mutual fund accounts that started with a modest deposit and were only being funded with $25 or $50 per month would grow into notable balances even after only ten years. It was eye-opening.

When you are only twenty years old and from a modest farm town, looking at six figures seems like a LOT of money; millions seemed like a dream! These people were rich! From all the investment summaries that I put together for folks, I learned that when your employer offers a 401(k), participate in it, especially if the employer is providing a match. An employer's match to your contribution is FREE money! Take it. The contributions you make into your retirement account are not taxed (pre-tax), so you are saving money by not paying taxes on what would be taxable income. Most people don't even miss the money they are investing and not using as take-home pay. If you don't see it, you won't miss it. Invest in your employer's 401(k) and take the free money! You will be thankful for it later!

The rule of thumb is that money invested into mutual funds should double every seven years. Working at Agnew Young & Associates seems like it was yesterday, but it was twenty-eight years ago. That is four sets of seven years! Jim Agnew and Carol Young started a 401(k) for me, and by the time I left the firm it only amounted to maybe $10,000. I have not touched those funds and have let them sit in that retirement account all these years. Time goes by quickly, and so that $10,000 doubled in seven years equals $20,000; doubling again in another seven years equals $40,000; doubling again in another seven years equals $80,000; doubling again in another seven years equals $160,000 today. That ten grand set aside for me back then has turned into six figures today and will double again in the next seven years, which will be very useful as I get closer to retirement. Thank you, Jim and Carol, for teaching me such a valuable lesson in investing.

Like most young people just out of college who are starting their first real job it is quite common to want 100% of your paycheck to go into your bank account to pay bills and use for fun money. I was fortunate to have worked for a small financial firm that really taught me early on (when I was living paycheck to paycheck) to set some money aside, even if it is $25 or $50 each month. Back then, I could have just as easily used what I was contributing to my new 401(k) at the hair or nail salon, on my wardrobe, for a new designer handbag, or on the weekends when I was out with friends. Spending money on the fun things in life is totally okay; everyone deserves a treat now and then (just like dessert). But making sure you are saving a portion of your hard-earned money for a rainy day is important for your future! There will come a time when you need a larger sum of cash: for a car, a down payment on a home, a vacation, or maybe even for an emergency. Don't spend all your money in the present, invest some for when you might need it the most. Make your deposits into savings or retirement part of your monthly budget.

Be disciplined enough to trade unnecessary spending for investing. It does not have to be a lot. Here is some food for thought; spend less on dining out and expensive drinks and use that money to fund an account that will give you a greater benefit in the future.

Today, spending on lavish coffee concoctions has become so incredibly common. Young and old alike often spend $5 to $7 every day on a coffee habit and they are full of sugary syrups. Financially and nutritionally unhealthy! Side note: if your coffee is more than 100 calories, it's called dessert. A weekly coffee expense is roughly $30, totaling $1,560 per year: maybe more! Make your own coffee at home. In five years, you will have saved $7,800!

Fast food, take-out, and food delivery services are also very prevalent today. You cannot drive by a fast-food restaurant and not see a huge line of cars just waiting to order their food. It seems there is a long line no matter what time of day you drive by. Fast food has become a habit, something we have come to rely upon for nutrition. And just like those fancy coffee drinks, it is financially and nutritionally unhealthy. There was a time when fast food was considered cheap, but not anymore! A basic burger combo costs over fifty dollars for a family of four. Making a healthier version of the same meal would save that family over thirty dollars! A survey by U.S. Foods reports that the average person dines out 3x per month and orders delivery 4.5x per month![9] How much money could you be saving by making simple and easy homemade meals at home? Do the math!

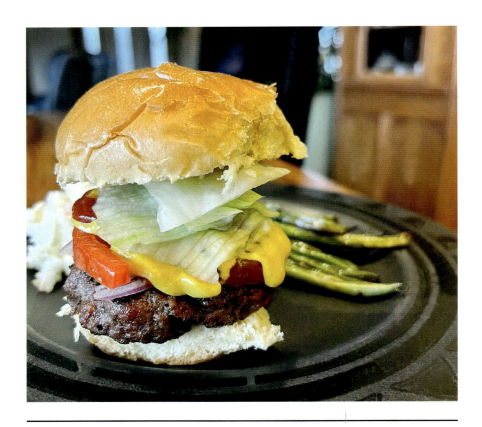

Fast-Food Take-Out
(4 combo meals)

Quarter Pounder w/ Cheese $13.31
Fries & Drink (each)

TOTAL for 4 Combo Meals: $53.24

Note: Costs based on 2024 data

Burgers on the Grill at Home
(Makes enough for 4, with leftovers)

4 ¼ lb Ground Beef Patties $6.37
6 Bakery-Fresh Buns 3.99
15.2 oz Bag of Potato Chips 2.85
32 oz Jar of Dill Pickles 2.59
28 oz Can of Baked Beans...........2.05
20 oz Jar of Mustard.....................1.05
20 oz Jar of Ketchup.....................2.05

TOTAL for 4 Meals + Time: $20.95

Turkey Burgers with a Kick

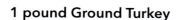

- **1 pound Ground Turkey**
- **1 Egg**
- **¾ cup of Breadcrumbs**
- **1 teaspoon Cajun Pepper**
- **1 teaspoon Sea Salt**
- **½ Jalapeño finely chopped (optional)**

Ground turkey is generally more affordable than ground beef. So, if you're trying to pinch a few extra pennies, give this great turkey burger recipe a try! Combine all ingredients in a bowl and mix thoroughly. Divide the mixture into four equal portions and shape into patties. Cook the turkey burgers on a grill or in a lightly greased cast iron skillet until the internal temperature reaches 165°F. Serve on a bakery-fresh bun topped with sliced onion, tomato, and lettuce. For a spicy twist, mix 1 tablespoon of mayo with 1 teaspoon of hot sauce or sriracha and spread it on the bun.

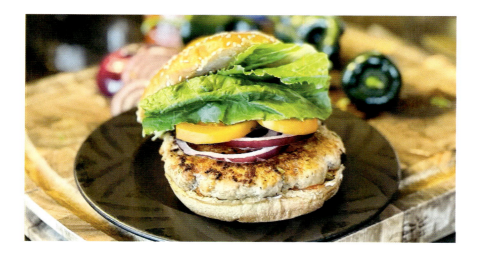

It is hard, especially when you are young, to think one year ahead, let alone ten or twenty years into the future. Believe me, the years go by faster than you can imagine, and before you know it, you are thinking about your financial future and when you can retire (hopefully early). Don't look back and wish you would have saved when you were younger. No matter what stage you are at in life, start stashing a few bucks aside here and there; it will add up quicker than you realize.

> **❝** *Gluttony is an emotional escape,*
> *a sign that something is eating us.*
> —Peter De Vries (1910-1993), American Author

With consumer debt reaching record levels, it seems that as a nation of consumers, we are losing the battle with temptation on many fronts. It is too easy to just charge things you want on a credit card or take out loans to purchase larger items. "Your eyes are bigger than your stomach" is not just a saying that applies to food. It is a saying that applies to material possessions as well. Consumers borrow way too much money, thinking that they can afford the loan payments without putting pen to paper. Never finance anything bigger than what you need unless you are 100% sure you can afford it long-term. Know your boundaries and avoid as much debt as you can. Debt is not fun; living paycheck to paycheck is not fun. If you get behind in paying your debts, it can be extremely costly in increased interest rates, late fees, and service charges. Debt piles up quickly, and before you know it, you're underwater. If you have loans, make your payments on time, and if you can afford to pay extra each month to pay off your loan(s) faster, by all means, do it!

Save up and pay cash for the things you want and need, if possible.

DOLLARS & SENSE

Avoid going into debt if you absolutely can. There are times when we need to borrow money, but borrowing money comes at a cost. Banks and credit card companies do not hand out free money for the sake of being nice. Loans are big business. Interest rates and financing options are important criteria when considering a loan, and they can make a big difference to your pocketbook if you are not careful. Let me provide a few examples:

Mortgage Interest: Let's say you want to buy a $250,000 home in rural Iowa. You have saved $25,000 to put down on the home, which is 10%. Interest rates are at 7.50% for a 30-year fixed mortgage. Monthly payments, including property tax and insurance, would be about $2,040/month. But let's say interest rates fall to 5.00% and all other data points stay the same. Lowering interest rates alone by 2.5 percentage points now puts your monthly payment at $1,675/month, which saves you $365/month. And, when purchasing a home, you must take into consideration property tax and insurance. These two expenses, on top of your mortgage, could add hundreds of dollars to your monthly payment. You should be aware of all additional expenses ahead of time to make sure you can afford your new home.

Auto Loans: Now, you want to buy a new car to put in the garage of the home you just purchased. The price tag is $50,000. The car dealer would like a down payment of $10,000 and offers an interest rate of 5.00%. Monthly payments, including taxes, title, and registration, would be $755/month. But, because you put all your money into a new home, you do not have any money to put down on that new car. With zero down, your monthly payments would be $944/month. That is $200 more every month for your new car, which will depreciate the minute you drive it off the lot. Unlike real estate, vehicles lose their value over time, so you need to be realistic about how long you plan to have a vehicle. Take the time to do the math or have someone help you. There is a real chance that you will owe more on it than what it is worth when you are ready to sell it or trade it in for a newer model a few years down the road. Getting financially upside down in a car can cost a person big time. And don't forget to factor in the expense of car insurance with your new monthly payment. You'll need it, and keep in mind that insurance costs can vary significantly depending on the vehicle you're driving.

Educational Debt: College education is another reason why many people go into debt. While interest rates on student loans can seem reasonable, and you can defer payments until after graduation, debt is debt, and payments will become due at some point. The average student loan debt is around $38,000, which equates to a $400-$450/month payment and $10,000-$14,000 in total interest paid over ten years. That can be quite eye-opening for any student graduating into the real world. Like with any other purchasing decision, price shop schools and think about the bigger picture when it comes to selecting a college or university.

Personally, I worked hard to pay for my education while I was going through school so I would avoid a large balance by the time I graduated, and yet I still struggled with a sizable portion that had to be financed through student loans. Maybe I would have done things a bit differently, looking back on it now after putting our daughter through college and having our son at the collegiate level today. While some of their peers are running off to state universities, big-name colleges, and private schools for $10,000 to upwards of $40,000 per year in tuition, we have taken a more conservative approach. If you are going to a "name brand" school for the college experience (football games, frat parties, and life on campus) or to simply say you have a degree from a well-known institution that everyone has heard of, think about where that puts you financially after you graduate. What type of degree are you pursuing and is it worth the price tag of the institution you are getting it from? Graduating with a business or accounting degree is a lot different than graduating with a degree in law or medicine.

If you are $120,000 in debt with a four-year business degree, your student loan payments will be $1,300/month for the next ten years of your life. If you choose to get a two-year business degree at a community college where the total cost for a two-year degree might be $10,000, you can avoid a good portion of college debt by being able to pay $5,000/year for two years of school and then finishing your four-year degree at XYZ University at $30,000/year for two years borrowing $60,000 vs $120,000. Even if you must borrow both the $10,000 for the two-year degree at a community college and the $60,000 for a four-year degree, your payments after graduation are $775/month (and $23,000 interest paid over 10 years at 6% interest), which is a lot more palatable than $1,335/month (and $40,000 total interest paid over 10 years at 6% interest)! Skilled trades might also be an option to avoid the cost of college altogether. Again, think through your options, have an estimate of what your income will be post-graduation with your hard-earned degree, plan ahead, and know exactly what you are paying for.

Most recently after 14 years of being a hiring manager and having hired a good amount of quality employees, I found that where any job candidate got their college degree never mattered. I never based my hiring solely on their college education, and neither did any of my counterparts. Having a higher education was important, but where that degree came from was never a factor. Instead, we placed greater emphasis on character, reputation, and personality traits, which often proved to be the most important factors in finding the right fit for the team.

The bottom line with any loan, whether it be for a house, a car, or a college degree, is to know your math. And, if you are not good at math, find someone who is: a friend or family member, a financial advisor, or your accountant. Run the numbers and never take a salesperson's word for it. The salesperson (or banker) that you are working with has a job, and that job is to sell you whatever it is they are selling (even a loan/financing) so they can close a deal and get paid a commission. Salespeople have monthly quotas, and most are out to make the sale to take home a bigger paycheck.

Know what you can afford and give yourself some cushion. Think about your annual income, consider other monthly expenses, look at the long-term, and factor in various scenarios. Be smart. Don't worry about what is popular or trying to keep up with the Joneses. Sometimes, it is okay not to keep up with them. I have seen many people in my time with pretty cars and fancy houses go bankrupt and lose it all. Just because you see someone with a lot of nice possessions does not mean that it is all paid for. They very well could have bitten off more than they could chew, and it will cost them in the long run.

With any purchase in life, big or small, you have choices. Bargain shop, watch for sales, price shop, and always get two to three quotes when purchasing a product or service. The more expensive, the more important it is to have one or two additional options to potentially save big bucks and still get what you want or need.

Cutting coupons is another great way to save some green. On Sunday mornings growing up, Mom and Dad would have the Sunday newspaper delivered. It was fat, full of news, interesting articles, comics, and loads of coupons. We girls would sit at the kitchen table before Sunday school and church and cut coupons for Mom, even ones for sugary cereal, though we knew it was unlikely Mom would end up ever purchasing them. Mom used coupons for the things we needed and stocked up on items we used regularly when she found a good deal.

DOLLARS & SENSE

Coupons are great, but like salespeople, their job is to get you to buy the product they are promoting. It seemed like coupons back in the day were straightforward with no strings attached, but retailers today have gotten more sophisticated and trickier with their offers to strive to outperform their competition. So again, apply simple math to find out if you are getting a good deal or not. For example, use this offer from a local grocery store: buy two 12-packs of soda at $9, get one FREE. Sounds amazing, but if the grocery store raised the price of the 12-packs of soda to make up the difference for the FREE soda they are promoting (which happens often), you are not really saving anything if the competing grocery store with no coupon has their 12-packs priced at $6. Make sense? You are still paying $18 for three 12-packs of soda, no matter what store you are shopping at. The FREE 12-pack deal was only to lure you in to shop their store. Consumers love FREE stuff, and they believe they got a great deal. Try to see past the FREE. Nothing is ever truly FREE.

Another grocery store example that illustrates the importance of knowing your math is advertisements for discounted items that people buy often; typically, it is milk, eggs, or bananas. The coupon (or television ad) might say bananas regularly priced at .68 per lb. down to JUST .28 per lb. Or one dozen eggs for only .99 (one dozen per coupon, per shopper). Consumers are being lured into the store to save very little—pennies on the dollar. You might be saving 40 cents on bananas through a store promotion, but if you spend $2.00 more on a pint of blueberries at the same store you bought the bananas, you're not really saving money. Instead of saving 40 cents, you're actually spending $1.60 more overall. It's important to look at the total cost, not just individual discounts. Buyer beware. Couponing has become big business these days and has expanded to more than just the coupons we used to cut out of the Sunday paper.

Couponing has turned digital. With today's technology, it seems as if every retailer in America has a perks card, offers membership rewards, or has an app you can download for discounts. When you really put pen to paper, most of the time the savings just are not there. It is all smoke and mirrors. The retailer gets your data, and then you get inundated with snail mail and spam to persuade you to buy more of what they are selling. Many times, we don't need any of it, but the deals look so incredible we cannot resist! Remember, consumers love a great deal. Don't give in to it. Most of us do not need to buy any more than what we truly need. Most of the time, we are not really saving any money by joining these "clubs" it is just a way for businesses to get consumer information for their databases. And, when you give your data to them for free AND spend money with them, they don't have to pay for your personal information AND they are making more money off you. Double win for big business!

The Mercantile in Fenton, Iowa, has long been closed, but to this day, I love to shop thrift stores and have taught both of our children to love finding a bargain too. It is a great way to save money, and I am fortunate that Mom taught us the art of thrifting before Macklemore made it cool. Go thrifting—you are bound to find some bargains, and you might even find a treasure or two!

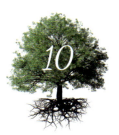

Harmonious Living:
Striking a Balance among Work, Home, and Life Demands

"Don't act like a chicken with your head cut off" was a typical expression growing up. You still hear the popular phrase to this day. Growing up my sisters and I literally knew what the saying meant because we really did cut chicken's heads off each summer. Our family butchered twenty or so broiler chickens (not egg-laying chickens; there is a difference) every year to freeze and eat throughout the year.

Fair warning: What you're about to read is a no-frills, behind-the-scenes look at life on the farm—specifically, chicken butchering. It's raw, it's real, and maybe a little messy. If you're not up for the details, now's the time to chicken out (pun intended). Otherwise, consider this your cue to roll up your sleeves and step into the gritty reality of farm life in this next paragraph!

Dad would take a hatchet, stretch the chicken's neck out over an old wooden stump, and "whack" its head right off. Simultaneously, as the chicken's head fell to the ground, Dad would throw the headless chicken's body by its feet up into the air, where it would violently flop around for minutes before it would eventually quit moving. Once the chickens quit moving, they were ready for the next step, dipping them in boiling water neck first by their feet. The quick dip in boiling water is to soften and open their pores, which makes plucking (pulling the feathers out) much easier and cleaner.

No matter how many summers we spent butchering chickens or how many times we witnessed the grim act of them losing their heads, each instance was a spectacle. The sight of a headless chicken flailing about is far from pleasant—it's downright unsettling. It's no wonder the phrase "Don't act like a chicken with your head cut off" came to be.

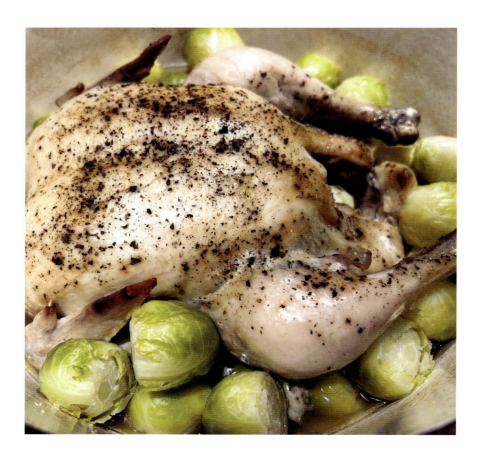

Whole Baked Chicken with Brussel Sprouts

1 whole Chicken

2-3 cups of Brussel Sprouts

2 teaspoons Sea Salt

1 teaspoon freshly ground Black Pepper

1 cup Chicken Broth or Water

And, if all that talk about chicken was making you hungry, here is a family favorite recipe you might enjoy!

Preheat your oven to 375°F. Pat the chicken dry with paper towels and rub it with sea salt and black pepper. Place the chicken in a roasting pan. Scatter the Brussels sprouts in and around the chicken. Pour the cup of chicken broth or water into the pan to keep the chicken moist. Roast uncovered for about 1 hour and 20 minutes to 1 hour and 30 minutes (roughly 20 minutes per pound), basting occasionally with pan juices. Use a meat thermometer to ensure the chicken's internal temperature reaches 165°F in the thickest part of the breast. Let the bird rest for 10-15 minutes before carving. Serve with the roasted Brussels sprouts and pan juices.

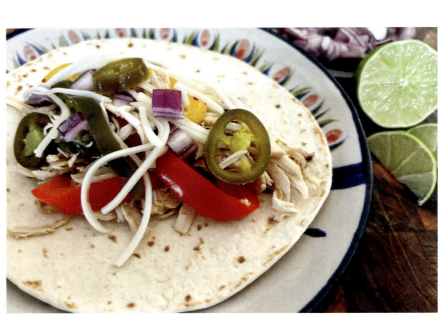
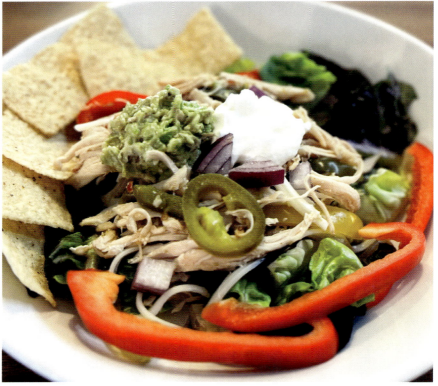

Colorful Crockpot Chicken Fajitas

- 4 Chicken Breasts
- 1 diced Jalapeno
- 1 chopped Purple Onion
- 1 chopped Yellow Pepper
- 1 chopped Red Pepper
- 1 chopped Green Pepper
- ¼ cup chopped Green Onion
- 2 teaspoons Sea Salt
- 3 teaspoons Chili Powder
- 1 teaspoon Red Pepper Flakes
- 1-2 cups Chicken Broth or Water

Place the chicken breasts, chopped vegetables, seasonings, and 1 cup of the broth in a crockpot. Reserve the other cup of broth or water. Slow cook all day, adding the remainder of the broth or water as needed to keep the chicken moist but not soupy. Once the chicken is tender enough, shred the chicken and mix well with the crockpot contents. Serve in a tortilla or on top of a bed of lettuce with your favorite toppings like guacamole, salsa, sour cream, and shredded white cheddar. If you have leftovers, add more chicken broth and some rice or noodles for a spicy chicken soup!

Sometimes, especially today, we humans can act like chickens with our heads cut off. With our packed schedules filled with long work hours, shuttling kids around, extracurricular activities, volunteering, getting to meetings on time, trying to get it all done—whatever your daily to-do list entails—I'm sure you've felt that frantic rush, worried that not everything will get checked off your list and there is never EVER enough time to accomplish it all.

Most of us struggle with feeling like there is not enough time in the day, and if you are an active parent, the workload can seem even heavier. Of all the jobs I have had over the years, being a mom has been one of the most challenging. Many moms must strike a balance between raising children, taking care of a home, making meals, managing schedules, working outside the home, and dealing with all of life's other demands. Dads do these things too, but the mamas in the world take on an awful lot, and it can be emotionally taxing.

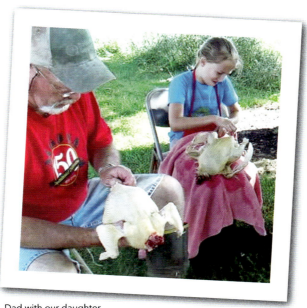

Dad with our daughter
Maslyn hard at work plucking chickens.

I wrote this job description a few years back and want to share it here in this book. If you are a mom, I appreciate you and recognize how hard it can be. If you are not a mom, you have a mom, and you know moms. So, please thank a mom for all they do. The struggle is real.

Job Description for Mother/Mom

Applicants should be well organized and have the ability to multitask. Must be willing to work overnights and weekends and be on call 24/7/365.

This is a voluntary position with no pay. There are no raises or promotions. Once you are hired, you are contracted to stay FOREVER. You cannot retire, resign, or quit the job. In turn, you will never be fired—no matter how many mistakes you make.

Experience in nursing, cooking, teaching, coaching, counseling, and supervising are beneficial. Storytelling and administrative skills come in handy.

Need to be a strong negotiator along with having a keen intermittent investigative intuition. Being a licensed lifeguard and having certification in first aid and CPR might be crucial. Mothers/Moms cannot be above serving as a taxi driver, maid, or garbage collector. Sleepless nights are common. And be prepared to sacrifice your serving of food to feed your hungry children. Temper tantrums and emotional breakdowns will happen. You will look ugly at times.

Ultimately, your job will be to produce little human beings and nurture them into independently productive adults who contribute to society. Being a mom is the toughest job a person could ever have. Most of the time, it is a thankless position. Regardless, you need to move forward and persevere.

No matter how undesirable the job description may seem, you will find the utmost joy, happiness, and fulfillment in your role. It is the most rewarding job a woman could ever have. Slow down and soak it in every single day. If you've accepted the position, you have been blessed.

Even at the age of 12, I realized how hard moms have it...

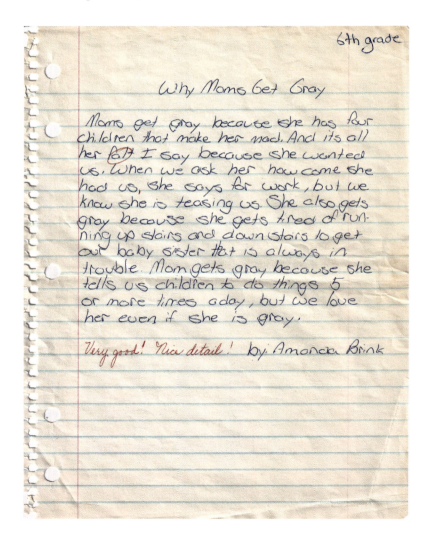

During my time as a mom, I have lost my shit. I'm not going to lie. The pressure of having to juggle it all has thrown me into a few temper tantrums that have made me look like a complete wreck; truly embarrassing when I look back on these ugly fits. I have acted like a chicken with its head cut off a few times, which does not do anyone any good. This is why trying to maintain a good balance between all our responsibilities is so important for our physical and mental well-being. We need to preserve a healthy balance to keep us from burnout and losing our shit.

When our plates are overflowing, it is perfectly okay to say "no" to taking on additional tasks. Sometimes, it is necessary to just say "NO." This might be volunteering for the PTA or driving someone else's kids to school, taking on a new work project or training a new employee, making a dish for the church potluck, or organizing a team fundraiser. Taking on more than we can handle is not healthy. When you say "yes" to something, you are saying "no" to something or someone else. Saying "no" sometimes only makes your "yeses" more valuable. Don't spread your "yeses" too thin, or they can quickly lose their worth.

Understand your commitments and what is involved: time, money, values, health, livelihood… Evaluate your obligations and prioritize the most important ones. It's okay to declutter your commitments by trimming the less essential ones. And if you find you have the capacity to take on more without compromising other aspects of your life, that's fantastic.

When we get overwhelmed with an abundance of tasks, it's common to delay starting them or to feel paralyzed by the sheer volume of work. A packed schedule can lead to procrastination. When we procrastinate, all we are doing is pushing tasks off until later. Those tasks never go away; they just stockpile until we decide to deal with them. Procrastination is something that can throw off our balance in life.

The things we procrastinate are typically the things we dislike the most. Maybe it is a tough conversation that needs to be had or cleaning and organizing a messy clothes closet. Regardless of the undertaking, tackling it head-on will free up mental space and help you avoid dwelling on it. Put the undesirable tasks at the top of your list to get them done and out of the way so you can move on to more enjoyable responsibilities.

Organized people are naturally less stressed and more balanced than those who are unorganized. Being organized may take some time upfront, but it saves so much time on the backend. Declutter and organize cabinets, desk drawers, closets, and pantries. Organizing our spaces and our lives helps us easily find what we need and reduces the stress and anxiety of searching for misplaced items. It is proven that tidy spaces cut housework by 40% and lower cortisol, the main stress hormone.

Another thing that creates stress and anxiety (at least for me) is running late. Running behind and being tardy gives me a great deal of stress, and so I always like to arrive early for meetings and events. Running late can also put undue stress on others too. I had a boss once who had a standing meeting with me every Thursday morning at 9:00 a.m. Every single Thursday, he would run late. His executive assistant would routinely let me know that he was running ten minutes behind or ask me if I could move our meeting back half an hour. Despite his position as my boss, his habitual tardiness showed a lack of respect for my time. Instead of sitting around waiting for him to arrive, I could have been using that time productively on other tasks in my already busy day. Being late doesn't just affect your schedule; it infringes on other people's time as well. I finally mustered up enough guts to tell him how his lateness was affecting my schedule (and my sanity). Thankfully, he understood my perspective, was made aware of how his tardiness was affecting me, apologized, and was on time for our weekly meeting from then on.

Time is a valuable resource for everyone, and being punctual demonstrates respect for others and their schedules. Plan ahead to ensure you're on time—not just for your own sake, but also for those who depend on you.

There are a million excuses for running late, and one that I have heard often (and used myself) is car trouble. So, make sure your vehicles have been serviced, have enough air in the tires, and have gas in the tank to avoid impromptu car issues or an unexpected empty tank that could keep you from getting to where you must go. I can't count how many times I've driven past a gas station on my way home, knowing the tank is on 'E,' convincing myself, "I'll fill it up tomorrow." By morning, I've forgotten, and that unexpected stop for gas on the way to work ends up making me a few minutes late, starting the day off on the wrong foot.

Just as keeping your car fueled keeps you on track, fueling your body properly ensures you stay energized and ready for whatever lies ahead. Meal prepping is a great way to save time and stay organized. Plan your meals for the week—or at least for the next day—to keep yourself on track and avoid unnecessary delays. As a Wellness Coach, I recommend meal prepping to all my clients. Not only does it save people from grabbing unhealthy convenience foods when they are hangry, but it saves them time during a busy work week by having healthy options available to them for meals and snacks. An easy way to meal prep is learning to love leftovers. If you are making one meal, make extra for the next day. It does not take any more time to cook an extra chicken breast or two, make a double batch of spaghetti, or roast a huge pan of vegetables. Leftovers are great to have on hand for later in the week, or if you are creative, you can use leftovers to make something new the next day. For example, chicken breasts can be turned into chicken quesadillas, chicken soup, chicken salad, or sliced and put on top of a beautiful spinach salad.

For those who order in, get takeout, or dine out for lunch, take a moment to reflect on the time involved in the entire process. The decision-making alone can sometimes feel like it takes forever. First, we decide what we're in the mood to eat, then figure out where to buy it from. After that, we either wait for delivery or take additional time to get to the restaurant, deal with waiting in line, traffic, and inevitable delays—all of which can easily add up to an hour or two each day!

Getting your food from a fast food or dine-in restaurant might seem like a convenience, but generally, it takes more time than preparing your own food for the week. Plus, unplanned meals and impromptu food choices are some of the biggest reasons we sabotage our own diets. By preplanning and prepping our meals ahead of time, we save time and money and are a lot healthier for it over time.

Deciding what to eat is one thing but choosing what to wear can be a whole different setback. Decisions and unexpected delays can all be avoided with a little planning head. I am sure we have all run late due to an issue with clothing. Whether it's your personal wardrobe, school attire, or a child's uniform, we've all experienced the frustration of being ready to head out the door by a certain time only to realize that a piece of clothing we need is missing or not clean.

Having your clothes and shoes in their proper dresser drawer or closet makes a hectic morning much more manageable. Keep laundry clean, folded, and put in its place. Delegate chores to family members to spread the load (no pun intended). Allow others to help you so the whole household is better organized and runs smoothly. The story below is a great example of delegating that I have shared many times. The story and lessons within it really seem to resonate with others.

Don't Refold the Towels

"Don't refold the towels" is a saying I came up with for myself after a few years of marriage. After complaining about how much work I did around the house and how much help I was not getting with the household chores, my hubby took it upon himself to fold the laundry one day to help me out. As I looked at the piles of neatly folded clothes on the floor, I noticed that he totally folded the towels the "wrong way." Being a very particular person, I took it upon myself to refold them the "right way" so they would fit the way I wanted them to into the hall closet.

My husband, Josh, immediately questioned, "Why did I even bother if you were going to redo everything I just did?" He made a valid point. If I was going to find fault with his attempts to help me around the house, what would ever motivate him to want to assist in the daily household chores? Refolding the towels would only discourage him from ever helping fold laundry again.

From his perspective, it was a lose-lose situation. If he does not help around the house, I am not happy. If he helps around the house, and if it is not done my way, I am not happy. So why even bother. Refolding the towels was an insult to my husband, who was only trying to help me. My response was basically telling him that the way he folded the towels was wrong and unappreciated.

After being married now for almost twenty years and having two grown children, I have learned to appreciate everything my husband and children do for me. Even when the kids were little, they learned to fold laundry, too, along with other miscellaneous chores around the house. Everyone helps around the house, and that is the way it should be. After all, help is help. And I recognize the extra time it gives me in a day, which is so incredibly valuable. Sometimes, the towels do not look perfect, or the groceries and dishes are not where

I want them to be, but that is okay.

The whole point of delegating chores and asking for help is to make your life easier and to save you time. If the people around you are helping to their best ability, consider it a job well done. Don't insult or discourage anyone by "refolding the towels." In fact, compliment them and tell them "Thank you." After all, they are just trying to help, and that should be recognized.

Know that it is okay to admit we cannot do it all. Delegate to others and lean on the people around you: your coworkers and peers, friends and family members, your significant other, and even your children if you have them. Kids are never too young to take on responsibilities. Just like Mom and Dad assigned us chores as kids, such as washing dishes and gardening, allow your children to help. Chores shape character and establish a sense of structure and responsibility.

Having a consistent routine and structure supports us with time management, keeps us organized, increases productivity, and helps us achieve our goals. Structure benefits everyone and plays a key role in fostering self-discipline. If you have children, providing them with structure early on is beneficial for them, and it is an advantage to you too, making your life a lot easier.

One of the most challenging aspects of raising children, in my experience, is enforcing discipline. Discipline is hard because we all love our kids and want to see them happy, and human beings generally hate conflict. It's often easier to give in because it feels like the path of least resistance in the moment, or it avoids creating a scene in public. But over time, giving in and lack of discipline will make it much harder on the parent(s), will cost more time, create more stress, and will have adverse effects on children as they get older. Now that my kids are adults, I can honestly say that structure, routine, and discipline have shaped them into two very responsible and successful human beings. It was not always easy, but it kept our household running smoothly (for the most part).

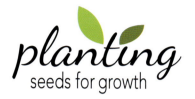

12 Hull House Rules for Kids
(and other guidelines)

---

1. Don't use food as a reward (especially sweets). Kids (and people in general) aren't dogs. Rewarding appropriate behavior, home runs, and good grades with food (especially unhealthy food) creates triggers. Triggers start bad habits.

2. Don't take away forms of exercise as punishment. Kids need to move and be active. Taking away school recess, sports activities, or going to the community pool should not be a form of punishment. Taking away apps on phones, video games, or social media seems to do the trick and is a better trade-off!

3. Don't use exercise as a form of punishment. Exercise should be fun and a celebration of what the body can do. Don't assign it to the negative.

4. Encourage trying new foods. Kids don't have to love them. But they should have the courage to try new foods, which could open doors to amazing new experiences they'll love forever. It can be magical, and they might just find a new favorite.

5. Create in the kitchen. Food is art. No matter what the age, there are simple recipes to get kids active in building their own meals. Get kids invested in what they put into their little bodies. Let them cook and bake. Nutrition is worth more to them when they're invested participants.

6. Limit snacking! Kids do not need to eat 24/7. Snacks are for long periods of time between meals when the body needs nourishment. Needing a snack during a two-hour movie, hitting the concessions stand at every sporting event, or wanting to eat snacks out of boredom IS bad. This creates triggers. Triggers start bad habits.

7. Limit video games!!! Video games turn kids into addicts and assholes if they're allowed to play them too much. We don't need more addicts and assholes! One hour a day IF all chores and homework are done AND if behavior condones. Maybe two hours on the weekends.

8. No cellphones at the dinner table (at home and at restaurants). Dinner time is family time. Time for valuable conversations. Don't let that opportunity pass you by as a parent. In the long run, your kids will appreciate those moments.

9. No videos in the car for trips less than an hour long. Again, this is valuable time to converse with your children. You'd be surprised what they divulge to you. Needing to watch a movie during a 15-minute drive is lazy on the parent's part. Don't be a lazy parent. Be an active parent. Use that 15-minute drive for quality conversation.

10. Go to bed! A regular bedtime is necessary to instill good habits from infancy. Sleep is crucial for growing bodies and brains. Be in your own bed at 8:00/8:30 every night—same time. Bedtime is NOT a negotiation. It should be a welcome time for much needed rest and a good night's sleep for EVERYONE and in your own space.

11. Electronics are put up at night. No phones/iPads are allowed at night. Phones get docked in the kitchen at 8:00 p.m. No phones in bedrooms. Bedtime is BEDTIME (not social media time, watching cat videos until you fall asleep time, making videos you'll regret time, or planning to sneak out of the house time).

12. Routine! Believe it or not, kids crave routine. A regular, normal daily schedule. Rhythm is momentum that smoothly moves you forward. Daily progress. Good habits.

Staying balanced requires ongoing adjustments and fine-tuning. Life is ever-changing, so be self-aware, stay mindful of your surroundings, and don't hesitate to ask for help when needed. Receiving candid feedback from people you trust can be incredibly valuable too.

Ask for new ideas and ways of doing things. However, anytime you ask for feedback, it's important to be prepared for honesty and understand that the truth is never mean. Truthful feedback is never intended to be hurtful; in fact, it can be very helpful if you are open to hearing the advice another person has to offer.

At times, we may persuade ourselves that we're not taking on too many responsibilities, that we're capable of managing everything, that our parenting styles are the right way, or that we've handled a challenging work situation correctly. We tend to justify (defend) all we do without taking a step back, looking at the bigger picture, truly evaluating the situation, and being open to other ways of doing things.

A few years into my sales career in television advertising, I thought I was really good. I was always a top performer and loved my job. Clients seemed to like me, and I had great customer relationships. There was one meeting in particular that I remember vividly. My boss, Dan, at the time (not the habitually late boss; he was later in my career) sat in on the client meeting as it was a larger opportunity, and so I brought in the "big guns" to help close the deal. After some small talk, I started the PowerPoint presentation and was working my way through the slide deck when I got a soft kick under the table from Dan. He was trying to get my attention. Once he got my attention, he took over the conversation, stopping my presentation. The remainder of the meeting was some back-and-forth discussion between all of us before Dan asked me to advance to the final slides of my presentation to end the meeting. After the client left, Dan explained to me that I was not letting the client talk. I was not listening. My agenda was the beautiful slide deck that I created, and that was the only thing on my mind during that hour-long meeting, showcasing every slide that I worked so hard on. Dan told me that I needed to listen more, talk less, and only give the client the information they needed. Sometimes, that meant skipping parts of a presentation to get to the point.

My feelings were hurt. I did not take the criticism well at all. The next day, Dan called me into his office to have a follow-up conversation about the client presentation that took place the day before and the discussion that he and I had afterward. After putting our next steps in place to close the business, which we were both confident we would do in the coming week, Dan reminded me about the constructive criticism he gave me and asked if I understood his perspective. He told me that "the truth is never mean" and that he was only trying to help me become a better salesperson. He was right. I was not a good listener. I talked way too much and sometimes even over other people. Ever since that conversation with Dan, I have become more intentional about asking questions, being a better listener, and talking less. His advice was beneficial in growing my sales successes.

To this day, I have the ultimate respect for Dan. He was a wonderful mentor, a tough boss, always fair, and always on time. Dan was instrumental in my professional development, offering various perspectives throughout our time working together. Dan's guidance contributed to my success in sales, which ultimately paved the way for my transition into a management role later in my career.

We all need truth-seekers in our lives to help guide us in healthy directions. Being open to different perspectives can offer insights, understanding, clarity, and the opportunity to grow.

❝ *Reality is something to be discovered.*
—Peter Schrag

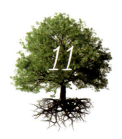

Connections Count:
Cultivating Relationships and Social Interaction

    The only electronic entertainment we had back in the day was the one black and white television set that sat in the corner of the living room and a boom box that I got from Santa Claus the Christmas when I was ten years old. It was accompanied by two cassette tapes: Michael Jackson's *Thriller* and Sheena Easton's *Strut*. The Christmas present was a notable upgrade from the eight-track stereo our family had in the living room. Cassette tapes were so compact and small in comparison to the collection of large and clunky eight-track tapes Mom and Dad had that consisted of great artists like Elvis, Neil Diamond, Johnny Cash, Linda Ronstadt, and Olivia Newton-John. Mom and Dad had probably one hundred or so eight-track tapes that were kept in two big heavy suitcases we would haul out every time we wanted to listen to music. My sister Sara and I would listen to "Ring of Fire" by Johnny Cash over and over and over again. We even choreographed a dance routine to go with it that we would perform for

Mom and Dad regularly. We loved the music on those old eight-track tapes and grew up listening to some of the best classics.

Regardless of how much we appreciated our parent's old technology, the boom box was one of the best gifts from Santa I ever received. It was silver with two large round speakers on either side and a cassette player in the middle with an FM/AM radio tuner that stretched across the top and right below the gray handle that went from one end to the other. I'd buy blank cassette tapes and sit in my bedroom for hours listening to *Casey Kasem's Top 40*, waiting for my favorite songs to be played so I could hit record and capture hit music for free. We had to be quiet while the songs were being recorded because our voices would be recorded along with the music. Even when we were as quiet as could be, there were times when I could not get a clean cut due to Casey Kasem talking over the intro to a song or a commercial that faded in at the end of a tune. Once songs were recorded, I would play and replay those songs to memorize the lyrics. Sometimes, I would try and write the lyrics on paper as best as I could understand them. There were only a few albums at the time that had the lyrics actually printed inside the cover. Man, I wore that boom box out! When it was not plugged in, it was with me on the school bus or outside. It took six D batteries, and they were replaced as often as I could afford new ones or steal some from a large flashlight that might be laying around the house.

The PlayStation came out along with the Game Boy handheld gaming system around the same time that I got my boombox. Mario Brothers and Tetris were the games all the cool kids were playing. But, like satellite TV (the huge round satellite dishes that sat in your front yard, so everyone knew you had a lot of TV channels), video games were luxuries, so our family did not have them. When it came to a lot of TV stations, Grandma Nita lived in the town of Algona, Iowa, and had hard-wired cable TV. It was a treat when we went into "town" to visit Grandma as she let us watch MTV, where we got a good dose of butt-shaking, tight leather pant-wearing, tattooed rock stars and rappers.

For the most part, we had limited digital entertainment, which left us more time to listen to my boom box, get creative, explore the outdoors, build forts, and congregate around the kitchen table. The kitchen was where we gathered not just to eat and to shuck peas, but our kitchen table served as the place we connected to talk, laugh, and sometimes play cards or a board game like Candy Land, Yahtzee, or Monopoly.

It is astonishing how our connections have changed since then. Technology has provided us with the ability to be connected all the time; phones, emails, text messages, social media, the internet… "Technically," we are more connected now than ever before, yet we have lost personal and meaningful connections with human-to-human interaction. Emotions and feelings are missing from the connections that technology has afforded us today. Even phone calls are becoming a thing of the past, with younger generations opting to text using acronyms and emoji-filled exchanges or sending Snapchat photos—often of their foreheads or other random, silly, and meaningless snaps—just to avoid breaking any streaks.

We had one phone in our house growing up. It was connected to the kitchen wall (and still is). And in my younger years, I remember only having to dial four digits to make a local call (within the city of Fenton). Local calls were free. Long-distance calls could cost an arm and a leg if we were not careful to monitor the minutes that we were on the phone by watching the clock that hung above the refrigerator. Being able to use the phone to call Grandma Nita or one of my friends was a privilege. I loved talking on the phone. But it being in the kitchen where everyone gathered did not provide very much privacy. And, looking back, that might have been for our own good.

Today, we are all on our phones a lot, but not necessarily talking on them. We use our phones for almost everything but talking. We use them as an escape, a way to pass the time or to avoid awkward silence when we are sitting in a room with others. Next time you are sitting in an airport or a waiting room, count the number of people who are not on their phones. You will be hard-pressed to find one. Or simply observe the tables at a restaurant when you are dining out and tally how many adults (and small children) are on their devices when they should be enjoying the company they are with. Our noses are constantly in our phones, paying no attention to who or what is going on around us. The days of eye contact and a smile from a stranger are fading. Literally laughing out loud in good company has been reduced to "LOL" and "LMAO" via text messages. True personal connections are becoming a thing of the past. Our connections are all on social media and that is how most of us connect. We are slowly becoming emotionless robots.

Smartphones' small size, ease of use, and portability make the risk of addiction even sneakier and more widespread. The consequences of smartphone addiction can be serious, affecting both physical and mental health and potentially leading to depression. Who would have thought that phones could create so many health issues?

For the parents out there, please avoid "babysitter" screen time for young children. It pains me to see young, small kids sit through dinner at a restaurant, church, or their big brother or sister's sporting event completely entrenched in a mobile device. Little ones are nearly 9x more likely to overuse screens when watching alone, and this creates unhealthy dependencies that may only be setting up toddlers for difficulty later in life. For instance, children aged 12 to 15 who spend more than three hours per day on social media face double the risk of experiencing adverse mental health outcomes, such as depression and anxiety. Research shows that screen time is "the main culprit" behind the skyrocketing rates of ADD, and the link between screens and poor mental health has become increasingly apparent over the last decade.[10] [11] The health complications from this technology are very real.

Kids are not the only ones affected by smartphones. Cell phone addiction affects everyone. Social media platforms consume so much of our time, whether we realize it or not. Individuals who frequently checked social media each week were 2.7x more likely to develop depression than those who checked it less often. And individuals with higher levels of smartphone addiction showed poorer performance in cognitive abilities, as well as in visual and auditory reactions. They also struggled with self-control, reported lower overall happiness levels, and had tendencies towards being procrastinators.[12] [13]

Permanent connectivity to our devices not only extends our working hours, it makes it very difficult to get away from the demands of friends and family. Instead of burying ourselves in our phones for work and entertainment purposes, we should take a break from technology and make real connections with real people face-to-face. I encourage everyone to challenge themselves and be intentional about establishing better connections to create stronger and more positive relationships by setting our phones aside. Put your phone down and engage in a real-life conversation with someone. Instead of staring at your screen, look up, make eye contact, smile, and ask how they're doing. Take the time to introduce yourself to new people. Compliment a stranger on their colorful shirt or mention how well-behaved their kids are in public. Remember people's names, and use them when talking to them, rather than just saving contact info in your phone. People love hearing their own name—it makes them feel recognized and appreciated.

> 66 *Recognize the universal power of a smile,*
> *for a sincere smile is courtesy in every language.*
> —Wilfred Peterson

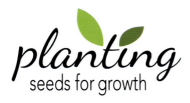 Reignite Your Personal Connections

Over the last few years, I have been trying to be more intentional about strengthening my connections (at least the ones I care about and are meaningful in my life). Here are some suggestions that might help you reignite your personal connections, just like they have mine:

1. Pick up the phone and call family and friends instead of relying on texting or emailing.

2. Wish people a happy birthday with a personal touch, rather than using a prewritten message suggested by Facebook.

3. Visit close friends and family—stop by their home or workplace with a thoughtful gift, like homemade cookies, a bottle of wine, or a book you think they'd enjoy.

4. Reach out to old friends or acquaintances you haven't spoken to in years, just to check in and say, "Hello." We all face challenges, and sometimes hearing from an old friend can offer a boost.

5. Handwrite cards, address the envelope, put a stamp on it, and send them by mail.

6. Take the time to get to know your neighbors better.

7. Make an effort to attend church in person more often instead of virtually.

8. Take the initiative to introduce yourself to new people you meet.

Human connection is a fundamental aspect of well-being for several reasons. Connecting with others provides emotional support. Engaging with others helps prevent feelings of loneliness and isolation. Strong social connections can buffer the impact of stress on mental and physical health. Building relationships and forming bonds with others create a sense of belonging to a community or group. Additionally, strong social connections have been associated with a decreased likelihood of chronic disease, decreased stress levels, better cognitive health as we age, improved immune function, healthier blood pressure, and a longer life.

Engaging with others, whether close friends or casual acquaintances, improves our well-being and nurtures kindness and empathy. Connecting with people in real, personal ways is essential for our health, but technology often replaces true connection with constant exposure to others' lives, whether we seek it or not. Through social media, we can "like" what people in our circles are doing with us, but we're also made aware of what they're doing without us. Social media highlights when we've been left out or excluded, making us more conscious of being invited—or not.

It is important to be mindful of the risks of social exclusion, as it can lead to significant consequences such as depression, anxiety, loss of identity, isolation, and withdrawal. Social exclusion is now recognized as a subgroup of bullying. Bullying back in my day was picking on someone in the hallways at school repeatedly and daily, taping signs to their back saying, "kick me," shooting spit balls through a straw (or a pen without the ink cartridge), or making derogatory comments about a person out loud so others can hear the smack-talk including the person being bullied. Today, bullying can take place online, both intentionally and unintentionally, and often goes unnoticed by teachers, parents, and even peers. While some bullying is directly aimed at individuals, social media can also create feelings of exclusion by highlighting what others are doing without you. Being left out, even without direct targeting, can have a harmful and lasting impact, making online bullying just as damaging as more overt forms of harassment.

Repeated experiences of exclusion can increase the emotional impact, potentially leading to the development of trauma. Over time, these experiences can carve neural pathways that register as deeply painful and impactful events. Seriously! Intentionally excluding someone repeatedly and aggressively with the goal of causing emotional harm is equal to verbal, physical, and cyber bullying. All forms of exclusionary behavior can have serious and lasting effects on the victim's well-being. Exclusion can, of course, happen intentionally, but I believe that it can be unintentional as well. When a person feels left out, and it is unintentional, I call it "unconscious exclusion." Below is a blog post that I wrote to describe how your connections can make you feel not-so-connected (or uninvited).

Unconscious Exclusion & Being Uninvited

"This is the best party ever! We are all here, but you're not because you weren't invited. We are having a great time…" These were basically the words used to caption a series of pictures (aka "snaps") of a giggling group of teenage girls. These snaps were directed towards our preteen daughter late at night, in her bedroom, on her cell phone, and all alone. She was purposely being left out of a slumber party that one of her so-called friends was hosting. Not only was our daughter not invited, but she was also being targeted via social media to make her feel even worse about NOT being included. Her feelings were hurt, and tears were shed. When I finally found out what had happened, pure sadness emitted from her entire little being. I felt horrible for her. My heart ached. I wanted to punish the little brats who made her feel so awful. Unfortunately, this happens more often than we think, especially in the crazy social media world we all live in.

Even if we are not being actively bullied into feeling left out, social media makes it very easy to discover when we have not been invited—not included. Most of the time, it is not as deliberate as the example of the slumber party, especially as we grow into adults. But it happens all the time. I call it "unconscious exclusion." Facebook, Instagram and Snapchat allow us insight as to who has been invited to dinners and celebrations, who all have traveled together as part of group vacations, and who has participated together in social activities over a fun weekend.

Kids get on Snapchat and can instantly see where their friends are gathered by looking at the Snap Map to see where the cartoon images of their friends are located on the map. When they see their buddies all group together in one location, and they do not get the invite, feelings are immediately hurt. Side note: this is also a great way to find out where the party is so Snap Chatters can flock in droves to the popular spot on the Snap Map.

Back in my day (decades ago), kids would pass out handwritten invitations for a birthday party at school. If you happened to catch wind of the upcoming celebration, you hoped and prayed that you would be the recipient of one of the coveted envelopes. If not, the party went on without you, and feelings were crushed. There might have been some scuttlebutt at school the following Monday. Social media obviously did not exist back then, so a plethora of braggadocios pictures that live online for all eternity were never posted, rubbing the "unvitation" in your face to make you feel even worse about not being included.

When you are the one scrolling through your Facebook feed and randomly come across a photo of your friends (or who you thought were your friends) all together having fun, and YOU ARE THE ONE missing from that photo, your stomach immediately sinks. You were not invited. You were not included in their plans. Why? Surely, they did not NOT invite you on purpose. There must be a good reason, right?! But still, you feel left out. Your feelings are hurt. You're sad and maybe even angry. This is "unconscious exclusion," or perhaps we can call it an "unvitation."

Maybe your pals figured you were too busy, did not have the money, or would not be interested in their plans. Perhaps they were trying to spare you from making a tough decision or having to decline their invitation for plans of your own. Or maybe—just maybe—they really did not want you to be part of their fun activities after all. It leaves your mind spinning, and your feelings still incredibly hurt. In a day and age where inclusion is a part of corporate policies and societal culture, it astonishes me that seemingly smart, educated adults in the working world are not conscious of the potential effects their "posts" have on others.

Kids can be cruel, but adults can come across as insensitive whether they realize it or not. 99.9% of photos posted on social media are the absolute best highlights taken from thousands upon thousands of snapshots in a day. They capture the best times of your life (or what you want others to know about and comment on). Dinners with friends, amazing vacation photos, touchdowns, home runs, beautiful prom dates, and new cars. We don't post about how hard marriage is, the stresses of being a working parent, or having to file bankruptcy. There are no posts about the arguments we have with our family or friends. No one posts about feeling lonely, depressed, or suicidal (all while their social media profiles display an entirely different picture of a happy life).

Parents never post about their kids fumbling the football, striking out, or placing last in a race. We never see posts about poor grades, temper tantrums, or not making the team. And never EVER do we see posts about the times kids get caught drinking, smoking weed, or getting busted for bad behavior.

There are way more strikeouts in real life than home runs, but we only hear about the home runs. We are all users of social media and need to remember that what people post is only a very, VERY small fraction of their lives, whether it includes us or not.

The next time you find yourself aimlessly scrolling through social media, ask yourself if you are happier because of it.

I listened to a sermon once that suggested that there should be five criteria for all social media posts we make, and ever since then I really try to abide by these guidelines:

1) True
2) Helpful
3) Inspiring
4) Necessary
5) Kind

Connections should be a positive experience. Though naturally where there are people, there will be disagreements. Any relationship you have can encounter negatively charged interaction. While disagreements are a natural part of any relationship, it's important to surround yourself with people who foster positivity. Associate yourself with people who encourage your personal growth. We have all heard it, and for the most part, it is very true, "one bad apple spoils the whole bunch." Surround yourself with individuals who share similar aspirations and values. If you want to have a successful career, a supportive family, and a strong marriage, hang out with people who have those same things. We have all had friends or acquaintances who drag us down, and sometimes, we need to think about cutting the anchor. Have the strength to part ways with relationships that hold you back from where you want to be and, instead, prioritize positive connections that promote advancement.

Because all relationships involve differences, and people often hold strong beliefs, one thing that can strain a relationship is when those beliefs are disrespected or infringed upon. We all have opinions, some stronger than others. Know your audience and never force your opinions or beliefs on others, especially if you expect to change their mind or if you know that it will start an argument. Being forceful and argumentative will likely never sway another person to change the way they think. Know that your opinions and thoughts are based on your personal experiences, just like their opinions and thoughts are based on their personal experiences. Know that you will never ever walk in another person's shoes and respect their views. No two people are alike, and no two people will ever share the very same opinion on something. Opinions vary widely from person to person, reflecting individual perspectives and beliefs that are based on their own life journey. As mentioned, where there are people, there are sure to be disagreements.

Since each of us encounters our own situations, you can never truly know if someone is facing challenges that are bigger or different from your own. Avoid making your problems seem more significant than others', as it can come across as self-centered and lacks empathy. It's important to recognize that everyone's struggles are valid. There are times in our lives when we need a shoulder to lean on, and it is healthy to allow others to help us. However, realize that the people around you have struggles too. We all carry heavy loads sometimes. Use your connections to share life's struggles, learn from each other's experiences, and support one another.

Much like forcing your opinion on other people, yelling and

screaming doesn't do anyone any good. Nothing positive ever comes from picking a fight or having a temper tantrum. Why waste your energy? Steer clear of aggressive arguing and never yell at someone in a conversation. You can influence others to see your way through healthy debates where both parties are open to hearing what the other has to say. Arguing and yelling often weaken your purpose rather than advancing it. Persuading others is possible and might even result in getting someone to come around to "your way" if done in a more palatable manner. Respect opinions and differences; we can all learn from them. There are times when we need to simply agree to disagree. And, sometimes, when we take a step back, we realize our opinions might be wrong, and we have opened our eyes to a new perspective.

> ❝ *Be the change you want to see in the world.*
> —Mahatma Gandhi

Just like arguing and yelling, gossiping often involves expressing negative or judgmental thoughts about others, which can create conflict and harm relationships. A common reason people engage in gossip is to seek validation or attention, often fueled by frustration, insecurity, or a desire to feel superior. Gossiping and name-calling can be extremely damaging, and we are all probably guilty of both at some level. Most everyone has been pulled into a damaging conversation about others. Nothing good ever comes of it, so why participate. The only thing that comes from it is maybe brief moments of entertainment, which are often at the expense of others. Gossiping never contributes anything meaningful to our lives. When we spend our energy negatively focusing on others, we divert valuable time and attention away from positively improving ourselves and building more positive relationships around us. Center your efforts on self-improvement, self-love, and extending love and thanks to those you are connected to.

Express gratitude frequently and acknowledge the kindness of others through regular acts of thanks. Gratitude is the one emotion that does not rely on any other emotion. You control it, and the more gratitude you create, the happier it will make you and others around you. Appreciate others and let them know it. Use your manners by saying "please" and "thank you". Practicing good manners has a significant positive impact on relationships and interactions.

Being a good listener also shows good manners and appreciation. Learn to be a good listener. I had to do this very early on in my career. For some of us, it is a difficult task. It can be hard to pay attention and difficult not to interject opinions and thoughts into conversations by interrupting and talking over people. Listen and allow people to finish what they are saying before you respond. Being a good listener requires positive body language, so be aware of your body language and facial expressions. Lean forward, avoid distractions (like your cell phone), make good eye contact, and actively listen. Be intentional about giving others your time and attention.

Helping others is another great way to foster positive connections and build meaningful relationships. Most people love to help; it makes us feel good. And being kind and generous is linked to better health. Helping is healthy, and it translates into happiness. Happiness comes from recognizing our strengths and talents and using them to improve our lives, positively impact others, and perhaps even contribute to making the world a better place! Helping serves a purpose. So, lend a hand and offer to help another human being when you can. Be the bright spot in someone's day.

And, when you say you're going to help someone, mean it. Following through on your commitments builds trust and credibility with others. Always do what you say you're going to do and keep your promises. When people know they can rely on you to fulfill your commitments, they're more likely to trust you in the future. Keeping promises strengthens relationships by showing reliability with both personal and professional connections. Failing to keep promises can lead to disappointment, frustration, and resentment. Overall, doing what you say you are going to do is an important part of building strong, positive relationships that benefit all parties.

We come in contact with a variety of people every day. Some we might know well, some casual acquaintances, and some strangers. We all encounter those who only help us because it is their job; they get paid to help us. They might help bag groceries, mow your lawn, service the air conditioner or furnace, serve you a beverage during a flight, or empty your garbage cans each week. If you get the chance to thank these folks, please do. They need to be appreciated too. And always tip your waitress and/or waiter. Having been a waitress, you don't want the reputation of being a bad tipper, especially if you frequent an establishment often. If you receive good service, leave a nice tip. Make positive connections even with people you may never see again. Again, it is an opportunity to be the bright spot in someone's day.

Recognize the incredible power you hold to uplift others and leave them better than you found them, even in the briefest encounters.

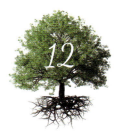

Unveiling Authenticity:
The Art of Being You

The same freshmen year that the used *Pepe* jeans incident happened, I experienced a few other run-ins with the same upper-class girls who laughed at me and my used designer jeans. I specifically remember one day during choir class. All high school grades 9-12 attended high school choir together. The freshman sat in the front row of the large music room and the upper class in rows behind them. During vocal warm-ups I felt my hair being lightly pulled once or twice and thought it might be because my hair was long and maybe was just getting caught in the seam of the metal folding chair I was sitting on. After a while, the very slight pulls on my hair became harder tugs, and I could hear snickering and whispering behind me. I sat there trying to ignore the upper-class girls, trying to be cool, and trying not to let it bother me. I could hear them say with disgust in their voices, "Her hair is so ugly," and "Look at her nails." It was the movie *Mean Girls* live and in living color, but only in 1989 before the movie came out. This was only part of a series of incidents that made me second guess my appearance; how I looked, my hair, my nails, the clothes I wore, and how I would ever fit into high school.

In the Brink household, there was a rule for all four of us girls: if we wanted to keep our hair and nails long, we had to be sure they were well-groomed and cared for. Mom made it very clear that maintaining long hair and long fingernails was a privilege that had to be earned, and both were our responsibility if we wanted to keep them. Otherwise, short hair and clipped nails would be the alternative. We all had shorter bowl-shaped cuts growing up, so I worked hard to have nice long hair and even learned to French braid it to keep it out of my face (if there was one thing that bothered Mom, it was hair that covered your eyes). And when I wore it down, I was sure to style it appropriately for the times. Grandma Nita was a beautician, and she started giving me permanents in junior high when I expressed that longer (and curlier) hair was the "in thing." Grandma Nita loved doing her grandchildren's hair. Once I got into high school, I started to pay a popular hair stylist in town to do my permanents. When it came to my manicure, Mom taught me how to file my nails. There were no nail salons back then, especially in small-town Iowa. I remember sitting at the kitchen table with her as she showed me how to round the edges of my nails with the metal fingernail file that she used. I made sure my nails were always perfectly manicured, along with being painted with bright-colored polish.

Looking back, there was nothing wrong with either my hair or my nails. In fact, I am confident that I had better hair and prettier fingernails than any of those girls who sat behind me that day in choir. But at the time, when I was only fourteen years old, they made me feel small and ugly. Their words and their actions stole a bit of my confidence. The way they picked at me really dug into any insecurities I might have had about myself. They were mean. They were bullies. And now, as an adult, I would not give them (or what they had to say) a second thought.

We all have insecurities, and most develop because we are way too concerned about what other people think, especially about us personally. We are constantly competing with one another and comparing ourselves to those around us, which affects our self-esteem. Back then, I was influenced by my peers' opinions and so-called standards. As it turns out, my guess is that their opinions about my appearance were based solely on jealousy.

Overcoming self-doubt can be an incredible challenge, regardless of where you are in life. It's a difficult process that often requires time, effort, and self-reflection. Instead of focusing on our positive attributes and what we are good at, we focus on what we don't have (or what people's opinions suggest we lack). Try to block out negative opinions and gossip that only come from other people's insecurities. Recognize where you are in the present, be content with, and embrace your unique qualities and strengths. We are all humans, and most of us are improving as we move through life. If you are on the right path and a path of growth, life will continue to naturally get better for you. Be patient. It takes a great deal of internal strength to be confident in who you are as a person. There is no need to be concerned about what others think of you, especially if they are meanies.

When you embrace authenticity, you set a positive example for others to do the same. Lead by example and remain true to yourself; being genuine can inspire others to follow suit and set a positive example. Use optimism to inspire positive actions and make a meaningful impact. Optimism and confidence are magnetic qualities that will not only benefit you but will help those around you and build them up.

Consider the multitude of negative thoughts and behaviors that surface when we seek approval from others or acceptance within peer groups, often just to fit in with people who may not align with our true selves. Be conscious and self-aware of these unfavorable tendencies. Recognize that the desperate pursuit of acceptance from others can undermine your self-worth and even lead to a loss of your core values. In many ways, this is a subtle form of self-sabotage.

It is so incredibly easy to be influenced into making choices that are not in our best interest—even if it is our own self that is doing the persuading. Our own minds can get in our way when it comes to making decisions. We can easily convince ourselves to skip the gym vs. going to the gym, sit around and watch movies vs. getting chores done, order a cheeseburger and french fries vs. making a grilled chicken salad at home, or sleep in vs. getting up and going to work or school. The path of least resistance is undoubtedly the easier choice. Healthier decisions may require more effort and offer less immediate gratification, but their long-term benefits are invaluable. Choosing the road less traveled demands discipline and mental toughness, but it's this effort that allows us to act in our best interest. Living a purposeful life takes intention and hard work, and the rewards are well worth it.

We can all be talked into making poor choices that go against our better judgment, whether we convince ourselves or whether we are influenced by our peers. Maybe it is being coaxed into having one more drink at the bar, knowing we should go home instead, persuaded to smoke a cigarette (or vape) when we know we shouldn't, convinced to go out for ice cream even though our friend knows we are on a diet, or encouraged to drive well over the speed limit to get somewhere faster even though we recognize it might be dangerous. It is so easy to be talked into doing things that could have negative consequences. What if we strived to set examples of courage by doing the right thing and inspiring positive influence in others to do what we and they know is right?

As we go through life, I believe (and hope) we become better at trusting our instincts. My advice to anyone, young or old, is to never EVER do anything you truly do not want to. I am sure you have heard, "If so-and-so jumped off a bridge, would you do it too?" The saying has been around for ages, and for good reason, because it is so tempting to do what others do, follow the herd, go with the flow, join the bandwagon...Do not sacrifice your values. Always make decisions that your conscience will approve of in the years to come.

If there is any regret in my life, it would be that I wish I never would have smoked cigarettes. As healthy as I am and all that I stand for today, there was a period in my life when I smoked! It makes me sick just thinking about it. My grandmother on Dad's side and my grandfather on Mom's side both died of lung cancer. I knew that cigarettes were bad. But in college, I started smoking anyway, but only on the weekends with friends and when we drank. I convinced myself that nothing bad would ever come from smoking occasionally. What was a sporadic weekend of a few cigarettes with some beers turned into a one-pack-a-day habit, and so I was a true smoker for the early part of my twenties. No one ever begins smoking, using alcohol or drugs, or gambling with the intention to become addicted. But it happens, and it happens very quickly when you hang out with people who do those things.

I heard something once that really made me think, "You are the average of the five people you hang out with the most." Seems silly to think about, but it is so true. Look at the people you spend most of your time with. Are they people you aspire to be like? Are they individuals you respect? Do they honestly have your best interests at heart when it comes to your overall well-being? Are they assets to you when you need support?...Birds of a feather flock together. If you aspire to be better than those five people, perhaps it is time to upgrade the company you keep.

It feels good when others accept us, and it is nice to fit in. There is no denying that. But never sacrifice who you truly are; always be you. Don't lose yourself in the attempt to fit in. Embrace your differences and dare to be different. People can still accept you despite who you are as a person, even if it means you are unlike them. If they don't accept you for the true you, maybe you don't belong in their circle. Remember that there are no two snowflakes alike, and every single one of them is beautiful in its very own way.

Genuine connections are built when you truly embrace and share your authentic self. Find people who appreciate you for your differences, quirks, and all the traits that make you unique and special. On the flip side, have you ever noticed someone who seems to change their demeanor depending on the group they're with? It's as if they're trying to fit in rather than being true to themselves. Maybe they dress in a different way, use language they typically never use, or their attitude and body language changes completely when they are around a particular person or group of people. We all have various circles of people in our lives; family, friends, classmates, teammates, coworkers, business associates... Being authentically you in every circle is a sure sign that you are the real you and that you are not pretending to be someone (or something else) based on the people you are around or the environment you are in.

Be self-aware and conscious of how you act in various settings and aim to be the real YOU all the time! Consistency is respected and reliable. If you need to change how you dress, what you say and how you say it, or how you act to be part of a group, you are losing yourself in the process of trying to impress others.

It's important for people to know they can trust in their authentic selves. Be genuine. Never lie. Always speak the truth. And when you make a mistake, have the courage to admit it. Don't make excuses and apologize if it is appropriate. Making mistakes and being wrong are natural parts of life and essential for growth. None of us are right all the time. Everyone makes mistakes. Own up to them, learn from them, and adjust.

Staying true to ourselves helps us face life's encounters with resilience and clarity, whether they're positive or negative. Life will throw us curve balls when we least expect them. How we deal with life's challenges shapes who we are; it builds our character. If you happen to have a bad day, find a way to move on. Don't let yesterday take away from today.

A great way to discover who you truly are is by spending more time alone. When you spend time by yourself, it gives you time without the distractions of others around you to think, be creative, and organize your thoughts. While connections with others are important, we should all strive to be independent. This does not mean that we eliminate people from our lives; it simply means that we take the time to teach ourselves to do things comfortably on our own, which builds confidence. I learned this valuable lesson early in my career during my early twenties from a dear friend whom I still admire to this day. It has been a guiding principle that has served me well ever since.

Build Resilience by Being Alone

"You need to spend more time by yourself," a friend of mine told me when I was about 21 or 22 years old. My workmate at the time (let's call her KJ) was roughly ten years older than me. I met her at my first-ever sales job. I really looked up to her and still do.

KJ caught your attention right away with her big blue smiling eyes, long lashes, and very blond Barbie doll hair. She was always dressed to the nines in heels and short skirts. KJ always spoke with confidence and demanded respect, though she was quite witty and had a raunchy sense of humor at times. She was not afraid to be a bit flirty with clients and knew that she was good at her job. KJ was an independent and established woman who lived on her own in a very modern townhome that she remodeled herself. Not only was she self-sufficient, but she was also extremely capable of anything she set out to do. That was very clear just by how she carried herself.

"You need to be comfortable going out by yourself. Try going to the movies alone," she continued to lecture me. KJ was essentially telling me that I relied too much on what other people were doing and lacked the certainty in myself to do what I wanted to do (with or without another person in tow).

I completely get what she was telling me now that I've grown from a young twenty-something to a fifty-something wife and a mother of two grown children. Maybe KJ's advice came across as a bit rough at the time because she said it in a very serious and mothering way. But it really stuck with me, making a lasting impression. I am not sure that I took immediate action on her advice, but I started to dabble in getting uncomfortable being by myself. For example, I remember a few months after that conversation with KJ, there was a wedding I was invited to. So, I did not ask for a date. I went solo. It took courage and felt strange at first, but it pushed me to have conversations with different people and make new connections, which ended in a very positive experience.

Fast forward five years or more…As my career in sales grew, I traveled quite a bit alone. I flew alone, ate at restaurants alone, stayed in hotels alone, and went on walks and runs alone in whatever city was my destination. And I thought about KJ's intelligent guidance to that girl in her young twenties quite often. Even though I traveled alone, it was still intimidating asking for a table for one at a restaurant, ordering a glass of wine, and eating chicken parmesan all by myself. But over the years, I have learned to love my time being alone. Being by myself has been therapeutic and has made me very comfortable with who I am as a person. I have realized that being by myself is totally okay. It gives me time to think, to read a book, or journal my thoughts and ideas.

Being alone does not mean I am lonely. There is a BIG difference. I have family and friends who I spend adequate amounts of time with. After all, relationships are a healthy part of life and very necessary for a person's social well-being. But, learning to be alone has provided me with the confidence to go against the grain sometimes. It has given me permission to not follow the crowd because it is the popular thing to do. And it has given me the power to stand up for what I believe in and be who I genuinely am as a human being.

Being alone builds resilience in so many ways. When you are by yourself you are 100% in charge of the decisions you make and the directions in which you are going. You develop abilities you may never know you had.

Six really great things that being alone can do for you:

1) Helps you expand your confidence in yourself
2) Keeps you from comparing yourself to others
3) Enables you to be observant and soak in your surroundings
4) Allows you time to find gratitude
5) Develops creativity
6) Offers you the bandwidth to think about and plan for the future

So, take yourself out on a date. Enjoy a glass of wine at your favorite restaurant, observe the people, and appreciate your surroundings. Hit a local coffee shop and read a book. Visit a public park and get in a good workout. Who cares what other people might think. Be confident to "do you" without any followers for support.

Be comfortable being with just you.

Thinking for yourself and being content with who you are is a beautiful quality to find within yourself. There are so many people in the world today who experience anxiety and frustration, being concerned that they are not good enough, which leads to self-sabotage, overwork, and depression. This is called imposter syndrome. We seriously have so much anxiety about fitting in and fear of not being liked that it leads to an incredible amount of self-doubt. We are often more attuned to other people's perspectives, not just to learn about them, but also selfishly, to be more liked by them. For instance, a 17-year-old girl shopping for a prom dress in today's social media-filled world will seek at least a dozen different opinions on which dress to buy rather than simply choosing the dress she truly wants. We all seem to place more value on others' opinions than on being confident in our own judgment.

KJ and I were introduced to each other at my first sales job, which was selling commercial advertisements on the radio. Since then, I established a very successful career in television and digital sales advertising. It has been almost thirty years since KJ and I met, and the advertising industry has changed a hundred times over since then. There is irony in the fact that I am a firm believer in the pursuit of independent thought and self-confidence, yet my career has been all about shaping public opinion for commercial interests in advertising.

Did you know that the typical adult is exposed to 3,500 commercial ads on any given day? These "persuaders" are designed to manipulate our behaviors. It's remarkable how easily we're drawn to trends and what we hear on the radio and see on TV and social media. Advertisers and marketers create ad copy to convince consumers to buy their products and services, some of which we need, most of which we do not.

It is important to resist becoming overly devoted to any brand.

Material possessions may briefly boost our self-esteem and fill temporary voids, but ultimately, they leave us feeling empty and hungry for more. You, not retailers or advertisers, should set your own agenda.

We are all very much influenced by the in-crowd, the media, social media, the fear of not fitting in, and the fear of failure. There are certainly moments in life when it's challenging to simply be yourself. Embrace who you are as a person. Be who you are all the time, enjoy who you are as a human being, enjoy life, appreciate others and their differences, and try not to worry about what others think. Slow down. Count your blessings.

Understand that you were created to be different than everyone else. It is by design. God did not make mistakes. Remember that you are like a snowflake amongst millions of snowflakes. There are never any two that are the same. Embrace the qualities that make you unique, that make you beautiful. I dare you to be different. Stand out from the crowd. Appreciate all your traits and characteristics. Simply love being you.

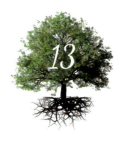

Forever Curious:
The Journey of Always Learning

We don't know everything (though sometimes we think we do), which is why it is important to always be curious and ask good questions. Just like little kids who are always asking "why" about everything. Why is the sky blue? Why do cats have whiskers? Why do I have to learn to read? Why do pickles taste sour…–Children are curious and are hungry to learn about everything. Just because we get older does not mean that we have all the answers. Have a hunger to find the "why" behind things. Keep an open mind because you never know what you might learn, which could make you smarter, wiser, more aware, and even more compassionate. For us to access this wealth of knowledge (behind the why), sometimes we need to get out of our own heads and open ourselves up to new experiences and perspectives.

Often, we convince ourselves that something is right or wrong because of our own beliefs and opinions. Don't let your own interpretations fool you. Politics is a great example of this. Democrats and

Republicans alike side with their party affiliation. But many of us share views from both parties and, because of our party affiliation, are unwilling to agree with (or even listen to) the opposing side. We can be so closed-minded because of who we identify as and who we identify with.

When faced with a situation, we tend to seek the answers we want to hear. People will keep searching for the reactions they want, no matter how many sources they have to go through to find the validation they're looking for. For instance, there are news stations that lean Democrat and there are news stations that lean Republican, so members of either party can find political perspectives that align with their own. And no matter which side you talk to, their news station is reporting the news correctly while the other station has it all wrong. Human beings gravitate to what is more palatable to their beliefs. We thrive on finding information that supports our own views to reassure us that we are right.

Similarly, the pharmaceutical industry can be just as controversial as politics. While some researchers may advocate the benefits of a pharmaceutical drug and promote it, just as many researchers may outline its risks and advise against its use. Whether it is politics, medical advice, religion, or relationships, often people will seek out the information they want to hear to support their own agendas.

Individuals love to be right, which is why we are so incredibly divided. People will argue simply for the sake of arguing. If you are one of those people who have a strong opinion and love to share it with the world, whether it is in person or on social media, please make sure you know the facts before you put it out into the universe. There is so much fabrication out there, and if you are not careful, you might be responsible for regurgitating bad information to the rest of us based solely on your strong opinion and wanting to be right. We are all too quick to accept what we see and hear when it aligns with our personal point of view, which is why taking a moment to pause and consider other possibilities is critical, especially in a world of misinformation.

As outlined in the previous chapter, humanity is made up of a very diverse group of people, and so it is important to understand varying perspectives. Our lives are all very different from one another: how we grew up, where we were raised, who raised us, whether we had siblings or not, our religion, the schools we went to, the peer groups who influenced us, the types of jobs and employers we have, our socioeconomic status, the color of our skin, our gender, our abilities or disabilities...

Often, we neglect looking at life with a multifaceted approach. We stop learning and become less curious. Perhaps it's because we become so comfortable in our own bubble, caring less about other viewpoints or even facts that might challenge our perspective.

We should always be learning from a variety of sources—a diversified portfolio of information. Our opinions and beliefs are shaped by a mix of personal experiences, insights from others, factual data, and sometimes even statistics—though these can also be manipulated to tell any story.

Our perspectives continue to change throughout our lives as we continue to learn and grow and as the world around us changes. It is important to ask questions and listen to others with purpose. Take the opportunity to be enlightened by another person's perspective and outlook on life. Just because a person has a view unlike yours does not mean they are wrong. You owe it to yourself to be open-minded to understand something new.

Prioritize learning and expand your knowledge on all levels. Always be learning. Actively seek out opportunities for personal growth. Below are some simple ideas to help you get started. Even though these are seemingly modest suggestions, they still might be uncomfortable or intimidating for some. But I encourage you to pick one or two that challenge you with something new while embracing the opportunity to have a little fun. Sometimes, you must push yourself out of your comfort zone to try new things. Who knows? You might acquire a better understanding of something you were unfamiliar with and discover something new you truly love!

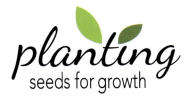

Expand Your Knowledge

1. Read a book. Instead of scrolling through social media, read a book. Make it a point to read one chapter a day. You are bound to learn something new, and it is better for your brain!

2. Explore a library or bookstore. Go old-school and explore the hundreds and thousands of books that are physically at our fingertips. Sometimes you come across subjects, titles, or authors that would have never entered your mind if you were not exposed to them.

3. Join a book club or start your own. Foster a love of reading. Book clubs are great for finding opportunities to share perspectives on books, explore new genres, and engage in thoughtful discussions that expand your knowledge and deepen your understanding.

4. Serve on a board or committee. Contribute your skills and ideas to a cause you believe in. It's a great way to get involved in your community, collaborate with others, and make a tangible impact on decisions that shape important initiatives or organizations.

5. Volunteer at a local nonprofit. Give back to your community. Whether you're helping with events, offering your expertise, or simply lending a hand, volunteering exposes you to new experiences while making a positive difference in the lives of others.

6. *Watch a documentary on something you are unfamiliar with.* Learn something new about a historic person or event, health, relationships, finances, or religion. The topics are endless.

7. *Listen intently to others and ask thoughtful questions.* Ask open-ended questions to find out more about people and their views. True engaging conversation is one of the most enriching experiences you can have.

8. *Invite a role model for coffee and conversation.* Find inspiration to learn from someone you admire, gain advice, and build a meaningful connection that could guide you in your own personal or professional journey.

9. *Take a class.* Expand your knowledge, develop new skills, and challenge yourself in a new area of interest by enrolling in a class or coursework.

10. *Job shadow.* Get firsthand insight into the daily tasks and responsibilities of someone working in a field you are interested in.

It's more important than ever to truly understand what's happening in the world around us and in the lives of those we care about. We owe it to ourselves to take a closer look and become better educated about the products and services we use daily to be certain we are making informed choices that support our well-being and values. We also owe it to ourselves to have a better understanding of the language used in fancy marketing. Afterall, over 90% of people are influenced by marketing. And marketers know that consumers choose products and services with emotion. So, feel free to poke holes in any claims that use compelling words convincing you and persuading you to buy something. Don't simply fall for clever marketing alone. If you are buying anything based on exaggerated advertising promises or flashy claims, you could be setting yourself up for disappointment. If you are buying solutions that promise a quick fix, you are very likely fooling yourself. Claims about looking younger, losing weight, or getting rich quick are often nothing more than empty promises and a bunch of bull crap. If they truly worked, wouldn't the world be full of youthful, fit, and wealthy people by now?

Words can be deceiving whether they are coming from someone's mouth, heard in a television ad, or seen on social media platforms. Words (and images) are powerful tools that can create hope, belief, and optimism. Think about the 3,500 commercial advertisements we see each day! Many of them really make us truly believe that we will easily lose weight, save or make money, improve our health, reduce the risk of chronic illness, and even sleep better. Advertisements use a lot of words like "may," "might," "can," "could," "some," "along with," and "up to." Here are some phrases to explain:

- "… may help you lose up to 10lbs in the first month, along with diet and exercise."
- "… can prevent heart attacks in some people."
- "… could reduce signs of aging by up to five years."

There is a lot of uncertainty in these statements, yet they are worded to give people hope that they can lose ten pounds, prevent a heart attack, and look younger. A fortune is being made on selling hope, dreams, and misleading promises.

Words are not just powerful tools used to advertise products and services, but they are printed on a lot of products we buy. Take, for example, cosmetics and hair products. These are some of the phrases that I found in my own bathroom:

- "100% of the daily hydration your skin needs to glow."
- "Gently nourishes for smooth, healthy-looking skin."

- "... soothe and calm skin."
- "... indulging skin with intense moisturization."
- "Age-defying."
- "Youthful vitality."
- "Instant firming serum."
- "... diminish the look of fine lines..."
- "Volumizing & hydrating formula."
- "Reduces the look of fine lines and wrinkles..."
- "... powerful antioxidants, rich nutrients to nourish hair and boost roots."
- "... high performance absorption..."
- "... creates a shield to protect hair..."

By the claims on half the products that I purchase and use daily I should look like a twenty-year-old model.

And what exactly is *100% of the daily hydration that my skin needs*? How do they know? And what precisely does *indulging skin* and *boosting roots* mean? And, *high performance absorption*, compared to what? All these descriptions sound amazing. "Calgon, take me away!"

❝ *Good advertising does not just circulate information. It penetrates the public mind with desires and belief.*
—Leo Burnett, American Advertising Executive

Numbers and statistics are also something you should scrutinize. Having worked in television for so long, spinning the numbers on ratings was quite common. Local ratings summaries and press releases regarding the latest ratings period might say, "Ratings Doubled at 4:30 a.m." If the station only had a .1 rating at 4:30 a.m.

before, and it grew to a .2, the ratings did technically *double*, but "Ratings Increased by a Tenth of a Point" does not sound as impressive as "Ratings Doubled." And oftentimes, you will see television stations promoting themselves as "number one," "having the highest-rated newscast," or being the "most watched." But you must consider the audience they are basing these claims on. Are the claims based on Adults 18+, Adults 25-54, Households...Any way you slice it, there is a large portion of the TV audience that is not included in their statement, and I am sure if added to the whole, it would change the headline drastically.

Surveys, polls, and research findings are other platforms that typically spin numbers or leave out a large piece of the puzzle. For example, corporate leadership might present a survey using employee results to their board as "70% of employees are satisfied with their jobs." But if only 25% of the employees filled out the survey, the 70% satisfaction rate is questionable. Let's do the math. If the employer has 200 employees and only 25% of employees (50 employees) took the survey, that leaves 150 employees who did not take the survey, and maybe for reasons that might impact the satisfaction rate negatively. 70% of the 50 who completed the survey is only 35 employees out of the 200 total. Those 35 employees reported being satisfied with their jobs, which is only 17.5% of total employees reporting overall satisfaction when applied to all 200 employees. That is a big discrepancy! The 150 employees who did not take the survey might have felt too intimidated to respond for fear of being demoted, not promoted, or even fired for giving their honest feedback.

It's important to be curious, think critically, and continue to learn. Don't just believe everything you hear without questioning it, especially in today's day and age. Look for information that is supported with facts and from reliable sources. And always have an open mind to new ideas and ways to learn.

Being curious and thoughtful, especially with a good foundation of knowledge, helps you better understand the world and the people around you. This is why a good education is so important. If you have kids in school, make their education a priority—it's one of the greatest gifts you can give them. As a parent you need to be curious about how they spend their time at school and to stay actively involved in their academic journey. Educators have less control than ever before over the curriculum they teach, how they teach, and how to keep students accountable both in academics and behaviors in the classroom. Teachers have one of the most challenging professions today. Between educational agendas, ever-changing policies, and out-of-control student behaviors, they are caught between a rock and a hard place.

Parents, be curious about what your kids are learning in school, how they are graded, and if they are getting their homework done. Ask your kids who their favorite teachers are and why. Ask them what happened at school today. You might find that there are curriculums, incidences and behaviors at your kids' schools that could really shock you. Open the lines of communication and allow your children to talk to you about what happens at school, both the good and the bad.

If I did not routinely ask my kids questions throughout their time in school, I would never have had a clue about a lot of things, such as my son learning about sexual positions (including oral sex) in health class in the 7th grade, or that kids get caught with drugs all the time in the bathrooms (and not just marijuana). What might be shocking to you as a parent can be normal to your children because they live it every day when you are not around. So, ask them questions. Listen. Have good conversations with your kids and be there to enlighten them with your perspectives on what they see, hear, learn, and even eat at school.

Because nutrition is such a key factor for children as they grow and learn, know what your school district is serving them for breakfast and lunch. I have found that school lunches are nothing but ultra-processed foods with little to no nutrition and filled with sugar. This affects a child's attention span, their behaviors, and how they develop. Their bodies and brains need healthy fats and good protein sources. A whole-wheat Long John and strawberry milk for breakfast and a whole-wheat pretzel with bright yellow-orange cheese sauce, an apple, and chocolate milk for lunch are not adequate daily nutrition for growing bodies. A donut and a pretzel (even if they are made with whole grains) are simply not enough to sustain them through the day.

Schools do not do a great job of teaching the importance of good nutrition in the classroom or in the cafeteria. If you have school-age children, I encourage you to check out their breakfast and lunch menus. You might consider having them take their own lunch. In fact, I encourage kids to actively pack their own lunch to get them invested in the foods they eat.

We should always be curious as to what we are feeding our bodies and our brains.

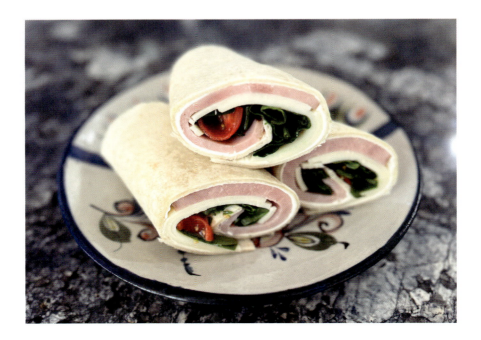

Wonderful Wraps

1 large Flour Tortilla

2 tablespoons Cream Cheese

4 ounces Sliced Turkey or Ham

Chopped Cucumber, Tomato, Onion, Lettuce, or Spinach

¼ cup of Shredded Cheddar Cheese

Spread the cream cheese over the tortilla. Not only is it tasty, but it protects the shell from getting soggy before it is time to eat. Layer the turkey or ham on top of the cream cheese. Add chopped cucumber, tomato, onion, lettuce, or spinach. Pick a vegetable or two to give the wrap some color and good vitamins. Sprinkle the wrap with the shredded cheese. Roll the tortilla and all the fixings up into one roll, cut it in half, and place it in a Tupperware® container or sandwich bag.

Healthy, easy-to-pack sides: cottage cheese, whole yogurt (watch the sugar and fake sugars), carrot sticks, celery with peanut butter, and orange slices.

Not only have I always talked to my kids about their school day and what they eat for lunch, but I contacted their teachers a few times every year to hear their perspectives and learn about any concerns they had. Supporting their teachers helps you learn more about your kids. You get some really good feedback from educators and sometimes even some nice compliments about your kids, which are always great to hear.

Our two children went to a large school district, each of them having roughly 550 students in their respective grades. Ever since they were in kindergarten, I loved attending parent-teacher conferences, which were held two times each year (once in the fall and once in the spring). Parent-teacher conferences were an opportunity for me to learn from their teachers about what my kids were good at and what they needed to work on. It also helped build rapport between me and their teachers to open lines of communication throughout the school year. During their junior high and high school years, I met with all their individual teachers, and I was always shocked by how few parents attended parent-teacher conferences. What a missed opportunity to ask questions and learn about the human beings you've created and are raising in this crazy world. Meeting with teachers is a wonderful way to support your children throughout their school years.

Stay curious. Always do your research. Take the time to ask good questions and explore the answers in all areas of life. Commit to continuous learning, and you'll be surprised by the new perspectives you encounter.

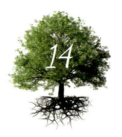

Mindful Navigation:
Being Aware in Your Environment

Our environment affects our lives and how we develop physically, mentally, and spiritually. Our environment is everything around us—our surroundings, the conditions, and the things that influence us. When you think of "environment," the first thing that might come to mind is our natural environment; the air we breathe, water, soil, plants, animals, and ecosystems. But we are also surrounded by what has been built around us, including buildings, roads, infrastructure, and urban spaces. Cultural, economic, and political contexts make up our social environment, which helps shape us as human beings. And our work environment has become a significant factor in how people function as discussed earlier in this book.

Our overall environment has changed substantially over the last fifty years. The modifications in technology, agriculture, big food, infrastructure, and culture since my time as a child are absolutely incredible. Everything from the houses we live in to outdoor spaces, the air we breathe, and the food we eat has changed because of advancements in technology and science, and how we, as human beings, interact with them. Some may argue that these changes make life easier and provide us with more conveniences and better opportunities. While that may be true, there are also real threats that lie within the advances we take advantage of today.

There are definitely some significant benefits we can all enjoy by using modern technology and science. The world has transformed into one that I would have never imagined as a child. I would never in a million years have dreamt that we would go from talking on a phone attached to the kitchen wall to talking on a cordless phone where you could see the person you were talking to in real-time on a screen. Back in the late 80s that seemed like something only possible in sci-fi movies like *Star Trek*. Or who would have thought that we would go from huge, folded-up paper maps that you would keep in the glovebox of your car to electronic maps that gave you directions on the very same device that you used to make phone calls? Or that kids in school would go from eating homemade chicken and biscuits with a side of cooked carrots to eating plastic-wrapped microwaved pancakes with the syrup baked right into them? Or that farmers would go from hours and weeks of manual labor in their fields to GPS driven tractors that drastically reduce the time needed to clear weeds from their fields?

I am not so certain that all these conveniences are for the better. The corn and soybean fields that surround Fenton, Iowa, no longer need anyone to manually walk or even ride up and down the rows, eliminating unwanted weeds. Round-up-ready seeds do all the work that a group of ambitious teenagers and farmers once did. Nearly half of all corn and soybean fields are sprayed with even more chemicals to eliminate unwanted pests and bothersome weeds. Fun fact for Midwesterners: Iowa, Illinois, and Indiana use the highest amounts of weedkillers containing glyphosate. For those of you not familiar with glyphosate; it is a widely used herbicide that kills weeds by targeting an enzyme that plants need to grow. While it's effective for farming and landscaping, concerns have been raised about its potential impact on human health and the environment.

Recently, while I was visiting my childhood home, I just stood back and took in the scenery, reminiscing about how it once looked decades ago, endless fields of green, gorgeous sunrises, and even more beautiful sunsets. Today in amongst the fields that surround those three acres I grew up on, stand hundreds (maybe thousands) of windmills; too many to count. The view outside the home where Mom and Dad raised us four girls is now littered with massive fiberglass wind turbines, all with blinking lights at the top of each one that stand out in the night sky. The red blinking lights that sit on top of these obnoxious structures completely distract from the pure beauty of the stars at night.

As I sat observing the changes in the landscape, there was a heavy mist that sat above the fields of corn. It was a humid summer morning. Mom and I were curiously talking about this heavy layer of fog that seemed to hover over miles upon miles of cropland when she made a statement that took me by surprise, "the humidity from the corn is full of chemicals." I never thought of it like that, but she was right. The air smelled a little like manure from the hog confinement across the road, which was normal depending on the direction of the wind, but it also smelled metallic, not like the pure natural air I remembered as a kid. The amount of chemicals in and on our crops likely evaporate with the moisture from the plants and, in that process, fill the air we breathe.

From Roundup® ready seeds to the abundance of chemicals sprayed on the crops that feed our livestock (which we eat) and go into so many industrialized foods we consume as humans; it seems as if the entire process of growing crops starts and ends with hazardous chemicals. Glyphosate is one of many chemicals being used. Roundup® (aka glyphosate) has been around since Monsanto introduced it to the market in 1974, but glyphosate itself has existed since 1950. Sales increased dramatically in the 1990s and have continued to go up every year thereafter. Glyphosate is used to kill weeds, but did you know that today, it is also sprayed on the crops themselves to kill the crops being purposely grown, so they are ready to harvest sooner than if they were left to die naturally? What!? This process allows the farmer to clear the field before the onset of unfavorable weather. It is done out of convenience in corporate farming.

Another fun fact is that glyphosate was patented as an antibiotic (kills bacteria), and today, it is found in 80-90% of grain-based foods we eat! It is marketed as being safe for animals and humans, but recent studies link it to cancer. It seems as if there is conflicting research about this widely used product. Imagine what it does to our bodies, especially our digestive systems. If it kills bacteria, it is killing the good bugs that live in our gut, the ones that keep us healthy. It lives in our intestinal lining and literally pokes holes in the gut lining, causing intestinal malabsorption and a leaky gut.

In mammals, including humans, glyphosate mainly has cytotoxic and genotoxic effects, causes inflammation, and affects lymphocyte functions and the interactions between microorganisms and the immune system. Roundup® is an herbicide (kills vegetation). Pesticides (kill pests and insects) that are used on crops are also linked to ear infections in children, fertility issues, and allergies, among other concerns. Between herbicides and pesticides, we are saturating our environment with a deadly duo! We are literally breathing in and mindlessly consuming chemicals every day!

These dangerous chemicals, along with many others, are found in the ultra-processed foods we eat. Industrialized foods are far from natural and are often loaded with additives that can harm our health over time. The food industry has come a long way to create food-like substances that appeal to our senses, and they want us to believe (through creative marketing) that we are eating real food and claim that it is even good for us. Big food hires thousands of scientists to essentially perform chemistry experiments to develop the best combinations of ingredients to get people to consume more. Enticing smells, mouth-watering flavors, and appealing colors are all part of the process to lure consumers in and get them addicted to the food being created in a lab.

On top of creating the most enticing processed foods, bioengineered food is also big business. Bioengineering is the process of changing an organism's DNA, which often results in foods that have been changed in an unnatural way and are not good for our health. These bioengineered food products can introduce new organisms into our bodies that can cause harm. Not natural! Our bodies simply don't biologically recognize the foods that make up much of our modern diet, as they are far removed from the natural whole foods our bodies are designed to process.

The American snack industry alone amounts to $114 billion in sales annually. If you are snacking, you are likely eating ultra-processed foods. Up to 71% of packaged foods sold in the U.S. are considered ultra-processed. 60-70% of the American diet is made up of ultra-processed foods. Research shows that even just one more serving of ultra-processed food a day can raise your risk of early death by 18%.[14][15] Excessive consumption of these foods that typically come in a box, bag or wrapper increases the risk of death. And if we are not dying from ultra-processed foods, we are getting fatter. Ultra-processed foods can cause people to eat about 500 extra calories a day, which may lead to nearly a pound of weight gain each week if not balanced out.[16] We are overfed and malnourished by consuming addictive food-like substances. More calories, more preservatives, more sugar, and more chemicals than whole, real food and far less nutritional value than our bodies naturally crave.

Consuming ultra-processed food such as soft drinks, fast foods, and frozen meals has also been linked to an increased risk of depression, which is most definitely contributing to the record levels of mental illness in our country along with being instrumental in the number of behavioral issues that children face today like ADD and ADHD.

Resisting processed foods isn't just a dietary deed; it's an act of soul-strengthening self-love. It's something you can teach your children, share with friends, and encourage in your community. This is why I encourage everyone to get comfortable in the kitchen. Educate yourself on the foods you and your family eat and take the time to create better and more nutritious meals that will serve as the building blocks for overall wellness and longevity.

Choosing natural whole foods is best, and if you can afford certified organic, even better. But know that just because foods are labeled organic, vegan, or natural, does not necessarily mean that they are healthy. "Healthier" might be a better word for most marketed health foods. Reading beyond the label is important if you are concerned with what you are putting into your body for nutrition. For example, one-third of "sports foods" are mislabeled as healthy. Powders, bars, shakes, and other drinks are marketed as being healthy for athletes but are not as nutritious as they claim to be. In reality, they are all processed foods, even if some appear to be more natural than others.

Today, the global energy and sports drink market is valued at over $159 billion in annual sales, with the United States alone accounting for nearly $14 billion.[17] Almost all have artificial sweeteners on top of artificial colors and preservatives, which are all harmful. "Fake" sugar products like Aspartame, Splenda, and NutraSweet can kill your stomach's good bacteria, making it harder to digest real food causing constipation. So even though you might be consuming "zero calorie" and "no sugar added," you could be doing more harm than good. But know that regular energy drinks' high sugar content can lead to insulin resistance, resulting in elevated blood glucose levels that can, over time, lead to prediabetes and type 2 diabetes. Either way, your best bet is to stay away from them. Go with 100% pure water. If you are an athlete and need electrolytes, you can easily make your own energy drink.

Energy drinks and sports drinks are not the only beverages that you need to watch out for. Commercially produced fruit punches and juice drinks conceal chemical additives behind their seemingly wholesome labels. Artificial dyes, flavors, and similar additives enhance their taste, appearance, and shelf life but are not healthy in the slightest. Food manufacturers have the goal to create visually appealing food and beverages that make consuming them enjoyable and fun for kids and adults alike.

"Whole grain" is also a label to watch out for. In the United States, food manufacturers can label their product "whole grain" as long as at least 51% of the grains are whole grains, which leaves me to question what is the other 49%? And, even if you are getting so-called whole grains in the foods you eat, remember that glyphosate is found in 80-90% of grain-based foods.

"Natural flavors" is another term that is used quite frequently, which really indicates multiple (sometimes over 100) individual ingredients that are used to create one singular "natural flavor." In some cases, the ingredients used to create alleged natural flavors in the things we consume today are not even truly natural in origin and are linked to serious health issues such as neurodegenerative diseases.

A well-known example of what I consider a misuse of marketing words is a popular breakfast cereal that has claimed for decades that

Citrus Charge Drink

2 cups of Water (or Coconut Water)
2 tablespoons of Lemon or Lime Juice
2 teaspoons Local Honey
¼ teaspoon Sea Salt (not table salt)

This is a great do-it-yourself electrolyte drink. Add all ingredients in a large glass and/or shaker bottle and shake well. You can double or triple the recipe and store it in the refrigerator to use as needed. 100% coconut water contains electrolytes and is a great way to hydrate the body naturally.

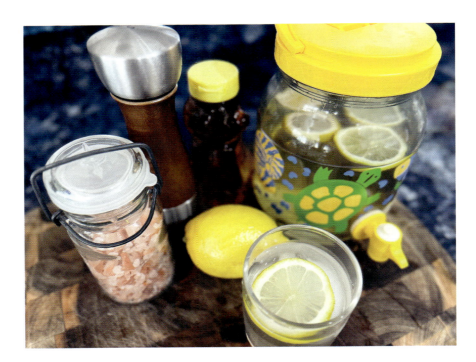

it *can* help lower cholesterol as part of a heart-healthy diet. Honey Nut Cheerios has been famously advertised using a cute cartoon honeybee in TV commercials to make this influential health claim and people buy (and eat) it up. But "can" is the key word; it "can" help with the stipulation (that is written on the box) that you are also eating a heart-healthy diet the rest of the day.

The box of cereal typically also displays target words like "gluten free," "whole grain oats," "natural flavor," and "real honey" in attractive big font on the front of the box that makes consumers feel good about buying and eating the popular product every day for breakfast. But if you look past the cartoon honeybee and the big, bold letters on the front of the cereal box and actually read the list of ingredients on the side of the box, you will find a different story.

Although whole-grain oats are the first ingredient listed, they are followed by sugar, cornstarch, honey, brown sugar, syrup, and salt. There is 12g of added sugar in every cup of Honey Nut Cheerios and less than 1g of soluble fiber. To lower your LDL cholesterol, the average person really needs 6-8g of soluble fiber every day. There is hardly any soluble fiber in Honey Nut Cheerios and a lot of added sugar.

When you understand the whole story, there is very little benefit in enjoying one serving of Honey Nut Cheerios and way more risk that lies in that box of sweetness. You might have a better chance of getting type 2 diabetes than lowering your cholesterol with your daily bowl of sweetened o's. If cholesterol is an issue for you, explore healthier alternatives that are a natural source of soluble fiber. Two great examples are adding a serving of black beans to a Tex-Mex omelet with 5g soluble fiber or spread one-half of an avocado on a slice of whole wheat toast for 2g of delicious soluble fiber. Both options offer more fiber and zero added sugars!

Tex-Mex Breakfast

2 Eggs made the way you like 'em
½ cup of Black Beans
½ Avocado
2 tablespoons Salsa

Scramble or fry your eggs in a skillet. Add a side of black beans and ½ of an avocado for extra healthy omegas. Top with salsa and even a little hot sauce if you prefer and enjoy!

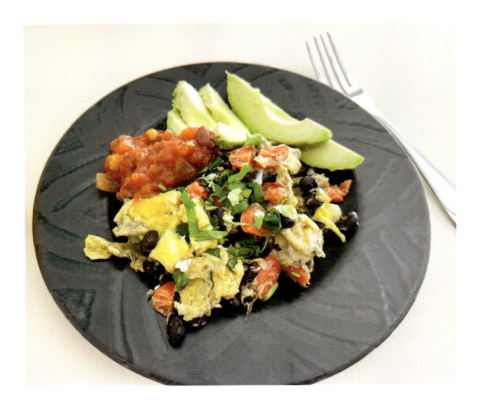

While soluble fiber helps lower cholesterol and controls blood sugar levels and is found in foods like oats, beans, and fruits; insoluble fiber promotes regular bowel movements and prevents constipation and is found in foods like whole grains and vegetables. They are both essential components of a healthy diet. Insoluble fiber acts as a "gut sweeper," increasing stool size, stimulating intestinal movement, and promoting rapid food passage through the digestive system. It can also dilute the numerous toxins we consume in today's American diet, such as heavy metals and pesticides, reducing their contact with the intestinal wall. Additionally, insoluble fiber helps to flush toxins out of the body more quickly.

Keep in mind that toxins are not just in our food, but the water you drink is likely full of them too! Along with chemicals from field runoff (here in the Midwest) that naturally enter the water we drink, nearly half of the tap water in the United States is estimated to have what are known as *forever chemicals*. Per- and poly-fluoroalkyl substances (PFAS) are invisible man-made chemicals found in our water systems, with high levels being linked to various cancers, reproductive issues, and adverse effects on immune function.

Microplastics, which can be found in many of the foods and beverages we consume, have also become a relevant concern regarding our health. Even though plastic does wonderful things, ongoing exposure to phthalates (aka plastics) is linked to increased risk of obesity, diabetes, endometriosis, birth defects in the male reproductive system, cardiovascular disease, and thyroid irregularities. It can also affect neurological development in infants and children, including ADHD, problems with behavior and aggression, as well as depression.

Just think of all the food and beverages that are stored in plastic. I remember the days when soda machines had glass bottles of soda for sale (they were also only 50 cents). There were no aluminum cans or plastic bottles. Now, everything is in some form of plastic. Almost all food and drinks are wrapped in plastic at every stage—from packaging to shipping and storage—before reaching the grocery store and eventually your kitchen, where leftovers are often stored and reheated in even more plastic. I've often wondered whether all shipping containers and warehouses are temperature-controlled, and how the process of cooling and heating plastic-wrapped items might influence the leaching of microplastics into food and drinks.

On a normal day, the average person might start out by going through the drive-through for a cup of coffee, which is put into a plastic or Styrofoam cup (heating plastics only boosts the consumption of more microplastics from that hot cup of coffee we drink). The cup of coffee we just purchased might be accompanied by a cellophane-wrapped pastry. We either drink out of a reusable plastic water bottle all day long or drink beverages from plastic bottles. For lunch, we use plastic silverware from the takeout restaurant to eat the food that is placed in a Styrofoam container. And, for dinner, we might try and eat healthy by cooking some chicken breasts, which have been placed on a Styrofoam plate and covered in plastic wrap, along with some frozen vegetables that we can microwave (in their own plastic bag for convenience) and store-bought bread that has also been bagged in plastic.

Not only do we consume microplastics, but think about the plastic in our homes, our offices, and our cars that we are exposed to every hour of every day. The amount of plastic we use and encounter on a daily basis is insurmountable. We have no idea! Something as simple as a plastic cutting board is prone to developing knife marks that release plastic particles into our food. And there are billions of used plastic toothpaste tubes that are sitting in the ground right now, taking hundreds of years to break down into smaller pieces of toxic plastic that leach into the ecosystem.

High levels of the industrial chemical bisphenol A (BPA) are found in women's activewear, from sports bras to leggings, exposing individuals to up to 40x the safe limit of the chemical BPA. We are wearing and sweating in toxic clothing! There are even pollutants that are designed to keep us safe like the flame-retardant chemicals used in the interior of vehicles. Although they have a good purpose, they release harmful chemicals into the cabin air.

Back in the day, when we would go asparagus hunting, all of the windows in the car would be down for a few reasons: 1) the vehicle was packed full of people who needed fresh air, 2) having the windows down provided us a better view for spotting asparagus, and 3) it was the only form of trying to stay cool on warm days. Plus, breathing in the fresh country air was part of enjoying nature.

Our cars back then did not have air conditioning, and you had to crank the windows down by hand. Air-conditioning was only available in newer vehicles, and central air-conditioning in homes was fairly new. I remember the day we finally got a window-unit air conditioner installed in our kitchen (even though Dad was against it). He was adamant that air conditioning was not healthy and was taking away his fresh air. But Mom was thrilled once the kitchen was air-conditioned as it meant that working in the kitchen could be done without sweating like a pig and that meals would be more enjoyable to eat in cooler temperatures during the hot summer months. The kitchen was (and still is to this day) the only room in Mom and Dad's house to have air conditioning. The living room and bedrooms did not have any air conditioning, so we used big plug-in box fans to try to keep us cool at night while we slept. Some nights, my sisters and I would all sleep in one room on the floor in a neat row just so we could use multiple fans blowing across us to get as much of a breeze as possible. We would also use those big box fans as entertainment, talking and singing into the spinning blades to create funny sounds. We would even stick Crayola crayons and pencils through the grate to see if we could create some kind of reckless spin art on the blades. Most of the time we just ended up with broken crayons.

Today, all cars are manufactured with air conditioning and all new homes come equipped with A/C. Unless we are outdoors, we are continually breathing recirculated air. Today, 90% of our time is spent indoors! And while artificial cooling does provide relief from excessive heat and can even safeguard us against heat-related illnesses, excessive use can impair natural immune responses. Dad had a very valid point, even back then. Fresh air is best! Open your windows or get outside.

Not only are we inhaling and ingesting forever chemicals, but we are also absorbing them through our skin. Our skin, which is meant to act as a protective barrier, is constantly exposed to toxic substances. Through hair products, soaps, lotions, sunscreens, and cosmetics, we intentionally expose our skin to toxins, allowing them to be absorbed into our bodies through our pores. 56% of foundation and eye products, 48% of lipsticks, and 47% of mascaras contain high concentrations of PFAS (forever chemicals), which contribute to low fertility rates.[18] Aluminum, found in antiperspirants/deodorants, may elevate the risk of Alzheimer's disease. Our bodies are designed to sweat—it may not be pretty, but it's a natural and essential way to release toxins.

Additionally, several studies have confirmed that endocrine-disrupting chemicals, such as phthalates commonly found in synthetic fragrances, can impair fertility and are linked to an increased risk of breast cancer.[19] When we apply makeup, spray perfume, light a candle, or use laundry detergent that contains fragrances, EDCs (endocrine-disrupting chemicals) are released, facilitating hormonal disruptions. And remember that all of these products are heavily marketed and promoted to make us feel better; meanwhile, they are slowly poisoning us.

We have been trained to breathe in scents since I was a kid. For those of you who grew up in the 1980s and early 1990s, remember Strawberry Shortcake and those awesome scratch 'n' sniff stickers you would get on an A+ paper from your teachers at school? Strawberry Shortcake's smell came from ethyl and methyl butyrate. Ethyl 2-methylbutyrate is a fatty acid ethyl ester obtained by the condensation of 2-methylbutyric acid with ethanol. It is a constituent of the aroma of wines, strawberries, blueberries, and apples. It has a role as a flavoring agent, a plant metabolite, a human metabolite, and a fragrance. The scratch 'n' sniff technology was created by scientists at 3M through the process of micro-encapsulation. The desired smell is surrounded by micro-capsules that break easily when gently rubbed. The rub-to-release action breaks the micro-encapsulated bubbles and releases the aroma. Does this at all sound safe, especially for small children? Between all the Strawberry Shortcake dolls, scratch 'n' sniff stickers, and the scented magic markers that we all used and sniffed during art class, it's amazing we all turned out okay.

We all love good smells. Almost every advertisement for any type of cleaning product has someone deeply breathing in their lavender-scented laundry or the air after spraying a lemon-fresh disinfectant. Marketers are encouraging consumers to breathe in lemon-scented bleach, mountain-fresh laundry soap, or pine-scented disinfectant spray, and we do it! Despite their "clean" representations, many popular household cleaning products contain a multitude of carcinogens that are responsible for chronic respiratory problems, headaches, and damage to the central nervous system.

Clean is not a scent. Clean is the absence of dirt, contaminants, and all smells (including the floral and fruity ones). Don't let advertisements convince you that your environment needs to be filled with scented chemicals to feel "clean."

We also have been made to believe that killing all germs with hand sanitizers and wet wipes is an effective way to stop the spread of illness. Even before the COVID-19 pandemic, many elementary schools were disinfecting students with Purell before lunch, after each recess, and all classroom activities in between. Parents in our school district were encouraged to send each child to school each year with a bottle of hand sanitizer and a container of disinfecting wipes to share with their classrooms. Once the pandemic hit, the use of these products sky-rocketed and the demand for them is still well above pre-pandemic levels.

But, just like our gut health, there are "good bugs" that we are killing with all the chemicals found in these products. While we are attempting to eliminate germs, we are also damaging our skin, which is the protective layer of the body. After all, a disinfectant is a form of pesticide, and along with the drying effects of hand sanitizers their use can cause long-term side effects.

People had double the levels of quaternary compounds in their blood during the pandemic than before – likely because of the widespread use of disinfectants, which can damage supporting cells in the brain. "Quats" are commonly found in household cleaning products like Clorox disinfecting wipes, and they are strong enough to cause adverse health effects.

The chemical load in our environment is overwhelming. While avoiding them completely is difficult, we can strive to be mindful of our surroundings, reduce exposure, and limit contact with substances that may impact our health.

Other than trying to avoid chemicals in our food and drinks, cosmetics and hygiene products, cleaning products and air fresheners, and even scented candles, there are simple things you can do to make your environment a little cleaner and a little safer.

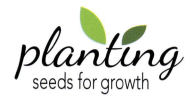

Clean and Safe Environments

- **Use stainless steel and glass.** Using stainless steel and glass water bottles and containers for your food helps reduce exposure to harmful chemicals like BPA and phthalates, which can leach from plastic into your food and beverages.

- **Don't use Teflon-coated cookware.** Teflon-coated pans can release harmful chemicals into your food, especially when the coating is scratched by utensils.

- **Cook in cast iron.** Cast iron skillets and Dutch ovens are durable plus using them to cook your food will add iron to your diet, which is a natural way to help treat anemia. You can maintain your cast iron's non-stick surface by keeping it "seasoned.

- **Do not microwave your food in plastic!** Avoid microwaving your food in plastic to prevent harmful chemicals and toxins from transferring into your food when heated.

- **Make sure you are cooking your food at safe temperatures.** Cooking at high heat creates inflammatory particles in food called advanced glycation end products (AGEs). AGEs can pass through the blood-brain barrier and incorporate into the brain cells causing Alzheimer's.

- **Avoid overloading the fridge.** If the fridge is stuffed with food, it can impede air circulation, leading to inadequate cooling and food preservation, which will increase mold and bacterial growth in the refrigerator.

- **Compost your food waste.** Composting will decrease the amount of household waste sent to your local landfill by as much as 35% in some cases. You can also repurpose food waste into homemade pet foods. Our family pooch loves carrot butts and broccoli stems, so I cut them up into pieces and mix them into his dry dog food for extra vitamins and nutrients.

- **Throw your garbage in the trash.** Do NOT litter. Pick up after yourself and your kids when in public places. This goes for restaurants and airplanes. I have always found it incredible that a flight attendant on an airplane can pass through the cabin at least ten times, and there is still a plethora of garbage in seats and on the floors. Littering is not good for the environment, and it shows a lack of kindness and respect for others.

- **Limit exposure to radiation,** such as from your TV and computer workstation. Excessive exposure to 2G, 3G, 4G, and Wi-Fi has also been linked to oxidative stress and cellular damage. Radiofrequency EMFs, most commonly released by cell phones, smart electronics, Bluetooth devices, and TVs, affect the vibration of charged particles inside the body. This has been found to cause oxidative stress inside cells, causing DNA damage, cellular damage, and inflammation in both human and animal cell studies.

- **Buy new bed pillows every two years** and wash your pillowcases once a week minimum. Both feather and synthetic pillows may contain up to 16 types of fungi, which can exacerbate asthma symptoms. And, when it comes to your pillowcases, they can harbor bacteria levels surpassing those found on a toilet seat by a staggering nearly 20,000 times after just one week of use!

- **Stay away from lead products.** Lead can surprisingly be found in ceramics, soil fertilizers, batteries, beauty products, children's toys, water supply pipes, and even foods and spices. In addition to reduced IQ, lead exposure stunts brain development in children.

MINDFUL NAVIGATION

- **Go scent-free!** Read labels carefully to avoid harmful chemicals like parabens and phthalates and choose certified products from reputable brands known for using natural and non-toxic ingredients. Utilize resources like EWG's Skin Deep Database to check product safety.

- **Skip the air fresheners and scented candles.** We love pleasant smells to fill our homes, but they often release harmful chemicals like volatile organic compounds (VOCs) and phthalates, which can contribute to respiratory issues, allergies, and hormone disruption. Enjoy a bouquet of fresh cut flowers instead.

- **Get outside** (or at least open the windows in your home and go for a drive with the windows down) and get fresh air. Getting fresh air boosts your mood, increases energy levels, improves concentration, and supports overall physical health by providing cleaner oxygen and helping to reduce stress.

As you practice mindfulness, remember to include your furry friends. Caring for our environment also means considering the well-being of our pets. Just as we scrutinize ingredients in our own food and household products, it's important to be aware of what goes into our pets' diets and the chemicals they encounter daily. Many commercial pet foods contain preservatives, chemicals, and dyes—similar to the ultra-processed foods we try to avoid. Likewise, cleaning chemicals and air fresheners can pose risks, especially since pets have their noses close to surfaces and frequently lick their paws. Creating a safer environment for them means choosing natural, pet-friendly products and being mindful of their surroundings to support their health and well-being.

If you have a dog, turn vegetable scraps into nutritious treats, reducing waste while giving them wholesome, natural ingredients.

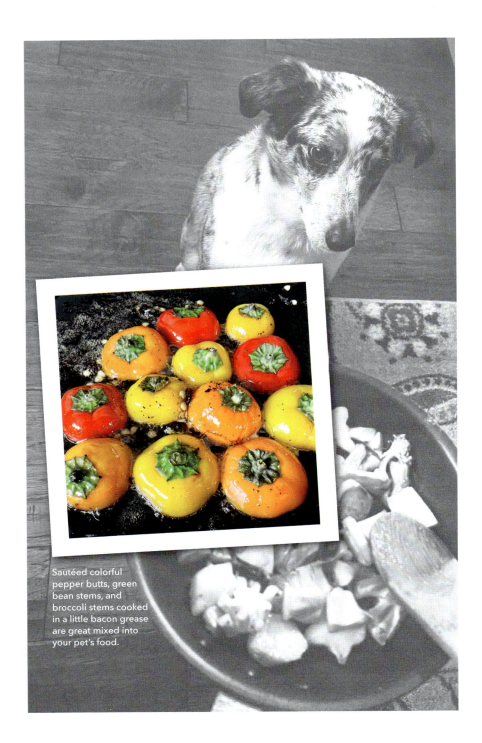

Sautéed colorful pepper butts, green bean stems, and broccoli stems cooked in a little bacon grease are great mixed into your pet's food.

If it isn't our physical environment impacting our health, our cultural environment will. Negative environments affect our overall well-being more than we realize. We have become so numb to a negative culture and divisions in society.

The human brain is wired to prioritize negative information, and we are drawn to adverse situations, which is why we gravitate to negative news headlines and harmful gossip/conversations in social media feeds. There is a lot of observed evidence that indicates humans tend to focus on, learn from, and use negative information from their environment far more than positive information. Negative things have two, three, or four times the impact of positive things.

In a report by the Centers for Disease Control (CDC) in July 2021, the two largest factors for COVID-19 deaths were 1) obesity and 2) anxiety and fear-related disorders. And we all gravitated towards the consistent 24/7 bad news that embedded fear and hate into our lives. In fact, we could not get away from it. Exposure to bad news increases stress. And stress can cause or contribute to increased levels of the stress hormone cortisol in the body and to increased risk of chronic illness.

Try to improve your environmental hygiene and eliminate pollutants from your surroundings for a healthier and more fulfilling life. Be mindful of the toxins you might regularly encounter and strive to remove harmful elements from all of your environments to protect yourself and your family. And don't forget to reduce the amount of negativity you encounter daily to help foster a healthier mindset and pave the way to overall well-being. Substances and material goods are not the only things that can be toxic. News, social media, and people can be toxic as well.

We've lost the simple awareness of being mindful of our environment and everything around us. With our noses in our phones, we miss an incredible amount of life, and we are also very lost. A friend of mine was telling me a story about their son who had just gotten his driver's license and was planning a solo trip to visit his grandma by himself with his newly earned privilege. Instead of using GPS, he just wanted to confirm with his dad some simple directions to get to his grandmother's house. He wanted to be sure where to turn even though the family had made the trip hundreds of times. The kid paid very little attention to where they were going or how they were getting there in his sixteen years of life because he was always either watching a movie on the in-car entertainment system or playing video games on his cell phone. It worries me today that so many of us are unaware of our surroundings because we are so engrossed in our smart devices. I hate to bring it up, but with so many school shootings and crazy shit in the world (all around us), I've had to remind my children many times to get their noses out of their phones when they are walking the halls at school, strolling down a bike path, or even shopping at the mall. Eyes up and ears open.

Pay attention and always be aware of your environment—always!

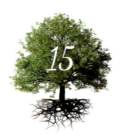

Guidance in Wellness:
Navigating Medical Advice with Confidence

When I was three (maybe four), I was lying on one of the cellar doors that lay at a tilt on the outside of the house. The old farmhouse we grew up in did not have a finished basement that you could access from the inside of the house, but instead had an outdoor cellar with two big doors that laid at a forty-five-degree angle from the east side of the house to the sidewalk on the ground. They were heavy doors you had to lift to lay open, and when opened, they exposed five larger-than-normal concrete stairs that led down to the dark, moist, cobweb-filled basement.

This might have been one of my first real childhood memories, and I vividly remember laying on one of the doors which was warm from the sunshine. The door I was lying on was closed, but the other door was flipped open. As I lay there sunning myself and playing with one of our farm cats, I must have tried hugging the cat too tight because she clawed at me to try and get away. Naturally, my reflexes had me involuntary roll away from the unhappy cat towards the opening and right off the closed cellar door straight down to the very bottom step. I don't remember much after that, but Mom said she heard me crying and screaming from inside the house and came to my rescue, finding me at the bottom of the cellar stairs in obvious pain.

A trip to the hospital would reveal a broken collar bone, which required an arm sling until it healed. I also remember Mom taking off my sling during bathtime to keep it dry and reminding me to be careful while I was in the tub during the weeks I had to wear it. I distinctly recall not being able to play the way I normally would in the old ceramic clawfoot bathtub.

Ten years later, when I was just starting high school sports, I would regularly have low back issues that would temporarily leave me bent over like the Hunchback of Notre Dame for a day or two. One day, the school nurse assessed me and informed me that I had scoliosis, a condition where the spine curves abnormally to the side. After dealing with on-and-off back pain, I started to see a chiropractor who discovered through an x-ray that my back, in fact, did have a curve in it. It was not confirmed scoliosis but perhaps a curvature that resulted from an injury sustained when I was young that was never addressed and forced my back to grow crooked. The day I fell off the cellar door always comes to mind as the culprit for my curved spine. If only we had gotten it checked right after the fall and had it corrected, but who could have known at the time?

My back gave me occasional problems from junior high school through my early thirties, but I refused to let it slow me down. I found that by maintaining a healthy weight (an extra five to ten pounds makes a huge difference in how my lower back feels), daily stretching, and strengthening my core muscles (all the way around), I could manage my back pain and eliminate painful setbacks. After starting CrossFit, which has only strengthened my core even more, and really watching what I eat, I am pain-free and cannot remember the last time my back actually "went out" or caused me pain, leaving me in hunched-over agony.

Keeping proper posture has also been critical for me in alleviating back issues. Good posture also has the added benefit of making you appear younger. Keeping your head up, shoulders back, and core engaged are key components to be mindful of whether you are sitting, standing, or walking. Repeated bad posture only worsens back pain by placing imbalanced force on the spine, which can lead to joint dislocation, increased discomfort, and, in some cases, nerve compression, disrupting a good night's sleep.

I am proud to say that I have avoided prescription pain pills and muscle relaxers, which were recommended to me a few times by doctors for my back pain. I have been fortunate enough to manage my twisted spine by eating a diet rich in anti-inflammatory foods and daily exercise. Taking good care of myself comes with a disciplined daily routine, which I have come to thoroughly enjoy. And it is most definitely better than being on prescription medications for the rest of my life.

> 66 *All diseases begin in the gut.*
> —Hippocrates, Father of Medicine

Physicians today are very quick to prescribe medications, whether it be to alleviate low back pain or lower high blood pressure, to treat asthma or address rheumatoid arthritis, to reduce the flareups of eczema, or to manage depression. Most of these chronic illnesses can be treated very effectively with diet and exercise. The sign of a good doctor should be how many patients they can get off medications versus how many patients they can put on medications (especially medications that are lifelong solutions to chronic illnesses).

As a wellness coach certified in nutrition, one of the first things I look at when working with any client is diet. So many chronic illnesses have a lot to do with what we are putting (or not putting) into our bodies. Skin conditions, high blood pressure, chronic pain, type 2 diabetes, mental disorders like depression and anxiety... When a patient is experiencing symptoms, it is a sign that there is dysfunction in the patient's cells. When you are experiencing symptoms of any kind, it means that your cells' needs are not being met or they are being overburdened with things they don't need. Prescription drugs, many times, are not a cure for chronic illness; they are only a way to manage the symptoms of that chronic illness for as long as you have that chronic illness. So why not get rid of the chronic illness itself?

In many medical schools, nutrition education is not a mandatory part of the curriculum. At best, it might be incorporated into other courses rather than being a standalone subject. However, there is a growing recognition of the importance of nutrition in healthcare, and some medical schools are beginning to incorporate more nutrition education into their programs. Regardless, nutrition education in medical schools today is very limited. A survey published in the *Journal of the American College of Nutrition* found that only 25% of medical schools in the United States offered the recommended minimum of 25 hours of nutrition education, with many offering less.[20] This is disheartening, especially considering the vital role nutrition plays in overall health and wellness—something that should be prioritized in medical training.

When choosing a family physician, be sure you find one who looks at the full picture, diet and exercise included. There are doctors who do a better job than others in exploring solutions that include a patient's overall fitness, which is the foundation for health. And there are some who are very quick to write a prescription which (again) only treats the symptoms the patient is experiencing; not getting to the root of the problem or finding a permanent solution. A friend once

GUIDANCE IN WELLNESS

jokingly told me that an MD stands for doctor of medicine, not a doctor of health. Laughing aside, this is something to seriously contemplate, especially when hiring a doctor to treat you and your family. If you prefer a more natural approach to healthcare, consider seeing a doctor of osteopathic medicine (DO). DOs are fully licensed physicians trained to focus on holistic and preventive care, emphasizing the body's natural ability to heal itself.

There are good MDs and good DOs, whichever you prefer. Just be sure you are selecting a medical professional who will spend adequate time with you, get to know you on a more personal level, answer important questions about your health when asked, and help educate you on lifestyle changes that could reduce the need for so many pills. Compared to other countries, U.S. citizens spend a significant portion of their lives consuming prescription drugs, with an increasing number taking five or more medications daily. In many other developed nations, there is often a greater emphasis on preventive care, lifestyle changes, and alternative treatments, leading to less reliance on drugs.

During an initial consultation, one of my female clients listed six different prescriptions on her intake form, which is something I have people fill out before we meet for me to do a comprehensive wellness consultation. The information that I ask clients to provide me with gives me a good amount of data about their current health, so I am prepared to go into our initial meeting with most of the information I need to help them effectively. Part of my responsibility as a wellness coach is to investigate anything that needs to be addressed when I create a customized nutrition and/or fitness plan for any client. In the list of medications that this female client noted, the first prescription was thyroid medication, the second was for high blood pressure, the third was for anxiety, the fourth was for occasional bladder infections, and she also took an occasional prescription for migraines and another for cold sores.

The thyroid medication did not mesh well with high-fiber foods and suggested avoiding calcium. The blood pressure medication listed kidney damage and headaches as potential side effects and suggested avoiding foods high in potassium (bananas, avocados, tomatoes, and apricots). The anxiety prescription that she was taking could cause difficulty breathing, and caffeine should be avoided while taking it. And dairy needed to be avoided while taking the medication for bladder infections. In building her diet plan, we needed to be cautious about high-fiber foods, calcium, potassium, caffeine, and dairy. And my observation was that perhaps the blood pressure medication was causing her bladder infections and migraines. Anxiety can cause cold sores to flare up. When I walked her through all of this during our consultation, she seemed a bit surprised and said, "My doctor never told me any of that." At least now, she is aware of how each medication interacts with the foods she might be eating and how each medication might relate to another. We are working on getting her off all medications, and I know we can get there alongside her physician's care.

Many medications on the market today receive rapid approval, often before scientists can conduct long-term tests to understand how the drugs impact patients' lives. While many new prescription drugs have demonstrated significant improvements in life expectancy and quality of life, some have not shown statistically significant benefits in these areas. For instance, certain medications approved for conditions like chronic pain or mild depression may offer symptom relief without substantial evidence of extending life expectancy or markedly enhancing quality of life. Despite this, the average annual cost of new drugs has increased by 53% since 2017. This should raise some serious questions about their true value for almost $378 billion spent on them every year in the United States, which is almost 9% of the nation's total healthcare spending, which is a stunning $4.5 trillion! [21] [22]

My husband and I are both very healthy, and very rarely have either of us been on any medication for anything, but when we started to have children (and got on a good insurance plan), I could quickly see how fast the doctors at the urgent clinics were in prescribing a medication for anything and everything that our family went in for. Most doctor's appointments consisted of a quick, impersonal five-minute exam that led to a diagnosis along with a prescription ready for pick up.

When our daughter was between the ages of one and two, she had a series of ear infections that seemed to be very persistent. The doctor put her on amoxicillin three times before recommending that we either try the next strongest antibiotic, Augmentin, or perhaps even think about having tubes surgically put in her ears.

Being a new mom, I was not quite sure about either option. My husband was all for tubes, as he explained that he had them put in when he was her age, and the ear infections were probably a genetic issue. I was still unsure, so I tried one last-ditch effort to resolve the ear infections by taking her to my chiropractor. My chiropractor explained that many little kids experience ear infections around the age of one or two because their bodies are growing so rapidly. During this time, their eustachian tubes, which connect the middle ear to the back of the throat, are still developing and can sometimes remain more horizontal or kinked than they should be, which prevents the tubes from draining properly, causing fluid to build up in the middle ear, which leads to pain and pressure. A gentle chiropractic adjustment can help realign the eustachian tubes, allowing the fluid to drain and relieving the discomfort caused by the blockage. What he carefully explained to me made sense, so we gave it a go, and after a few adjustments, she had no more ear infections. No Augmentin and no tubes!

Antibiotics are overprescribed in this country, with 47 million unnecessary prescriptions being issued each year.[23] Not only can we find antibiotics in our meat and dairy supplies, but Americans take an excessive amount of them when they are not needed. Antibiotics carry the risk of killing bacteria that are vital for the immune system to combat future infections. The over-prescription of antibiotics is fast-tracking the growth of antibiotic-resistant bacteria, which is only lowering our resistance to future infections. Consequently, 2.8 million antibiotic-resistant infections occur annually in the United States.[24]

One important thing to remember about antibiotics is that they do not cure viral infections such as the common cold, influenza, COVID-19, coughs, stomach bugs, and some ear and sinus infections. Antibiotics kill bacteria, not viruses. They should not be used for a cough, as they are ineffective.

And, speaking of coughs, most cough syrups contain frightening ingredients, including artificial colors, artificial flavors, and sweeteners, including high-fructose corn syrup. You can increase your cough-fighting powers naturally by mixing organic honey and/or fresh lemon juice with herbal tea. Honey possesses antimicrobial properties that do not worsen bacterial resistance, making it particularly beneficial for treating acute coughs in children.

Natural Cough Remedy

Water
1 Herbal Tea Bag
2 teaspoons Local Honey
1 slice of Fresh Lemon

Heat water and pour water into a mug, placing the tea bag in the hot water to seep. Add the honey and squeeze the lemon into the tea. Stir, sip, and enjoy.

If you have a stuffy nose along with your cough or cold, add four to five drops of peppermint oil to 8 ounces of hot water in a shallow bowl. Drape a towel over your head and breathe in the vapor for several minutes. This natural remedy can help alleviate congestion. We can become very dependent on nasal sprays and decongestants, so please use them with caution and only use them for 3 days otherwise, congestion can worsen, and before you know it, you are addicted and dependent on a medication to simply help you breathe.

Fast forward about ten years after all our daughter's ear infections. When our daughter was around twelve years of age, she started to really complain about not being able to breathe, and it was not due to a cold. She was always somewhat of a mouth-breather, and we never really thought anything of it; it was just the way she had always been. But, when her uncomfortableness and complaining got worse,

Peppermint Decongestant

Water
5 drops of Pure Peppermint Oil
Shallow Bowl
Towel

Boil water on the stove. Pour about 8 oz (or one cup) of boiling water into a shallow bowl. Put the drops of peppermint oil into the bowl of water. Drape the towel over your head and breathe in the vapor for several minutes. A drop of peppermint under each ear can also help with clearer breathing.

and she started to use and then beg for nasal spray daily, I thought it was time she went to see an ear, nose, and throat specialist.

After our initial visit, the doctor said that she had enlarged turbinates, which are long, thin bones inside the nose that are covered with a layer of tissue that can expand controlling airflow. He recommended replacing the over-the-counter nasal spray she was using on occasion with a daily prescription nasal spray. When I asked him how long she might need to be on the medication, he really did not know, the spray might work, it might not work, and he said that she might have larger-than-normal turbinates forever.

The possibility of putting our twelve-year-old on a prescription medication for the rest of her life was out of the question for me. So, I asked what else could be done regarding the enlarged turbinates. He said outpatient surgery to essentially cauterize them, which would deflate them in size and open her airwaves. It was a ten-minute procedure. We opted for the surgery. Even though there is risk with any surgery, the risk, in this case, outweighed the potential dangers of having our daughter use a nasal spray for an extended period (and maybe even forever to give her the comfort of breathing normally).

After she had the surgery, we got her home, and after she was settled in, I made her some scrambled eggs for her post-op meal. She exclaimed to me, "Mom, these are the best scrambled eggs I have ever eaten. They taste so good!" Apparently, the enlarged turbinates were not only affecting her breathing, but they were affecting how she tasted food too. Ten years later, she is nasal-spray-free and can breathe beautifully. I only wish we had had the procedure done years earlier had we known. She was not a natural-born mouth-breather after all!

From literally (and figuratively) one end to the other, society today is plagued by illnesses. When in doubt, do a gut check. Our gut health can be the culprit of many ailments we experience, from chronic pain to heart disease, skin conditions, and mental health.

GUIDANCE IN WELLNESS

Most diseases begin with the gut!

Today, it is estimated that 70M Americans suffer from digestive diseases like irritable bowel syndrome (IBS), Crohn's and celiac disease, ulcerative colitis, and gastroesophageal reflux disease (GERD).[25] Our gut health and microbiome are out of balance and messed up!

Our digestive system is required to help us digest and absorb nutrients and rid our bodies of unwanted waste. When our digestive system is not functioning, it can cause serious issues. Because our digestive system is hard-working yet very delicate, we need to be sure we are treating it well and with care. If we are eating ultra-processed foods, fried foods, added sugars, and loads of MSG, drinking excess alcohol, not eating enough fruits, not getting enough vegetables and natural fiber, and eating late at night, we are bound to end up with digestive problems.

One of the most common digestive diseases is acid reflux. Millions of Americans use antacids regularly to alleviate symptoms of acid reflux, heartburn, and other related gastrointestinal issues. The National Institute of Diabetes and Digestive and Kidney Diseases states that approximately 60 million Americans experience heartburn at least once a month, and about 15 million experience it daily.[26][27]

Antacids are widely used in the United States as a common remedy for gastrointestinal discomfort and acid reflux. And while you might think that acid reflux is when you produce too much stomach acid, it is likely that you are not producing enough. Stomach acid is critical for triggering digestive enzymes along with an escort "intrinsic factor" for B-12 absorption and managing local microbial populations. And vitamin B-12 plays a vital role in maintaining the health of the nervous system. Deficiency can lead to nerve damage and neurological symptoms such as numbness and tingling in the hands and feet, difficulty walking, memory problems, and even mood changes or depression.

I had a conversation once with a local pharmacist who was also a naturopath. A naturopath, or naturopathic doctor (ND), is a health-care professional who uses natural and holistic approaches to diagnose, treat, and prevent illness. This gentleman was retired, but I had asked him, how can you be both a pharmacist and a naturopath? It seemed to me that the two designated titles were conflicts of interest, total opposites. He explained to me that during the many decades that he was a pharmacist, he saw many customers/patients come in with medical prescriptions for gastrointestinal issues. After a time, he started to notice that the same customers/patients started coming in needing prescription medications for depression and anxiety disorders. That is when he began putting two and two together that the gut microbiome is affected by acid reducers, acid neutralizers, and heartburn relief tablets. And that these medications have a direct correlation through the gut/brain axis to a person's mental health.

After this realization, he became determined to assist people using natural and holistic approaches whenever possible, aiming to avoid the cascade of medication overload and its subsequent side effects. He observed how one medication often leads to another, creating a cycle of dependency, potential harm, and more medication! Thankfully this healthcare professional found a way to align his philosophies to a value system not guided by profits!

Mental illness is at an all-time high. Antidepressants are among the most prescribed medications in the United States. According to data from the National Center for Health Statistics (NCHS), the use of antidepressants has been steadily increasing over the past few decades.[28][29] A study published in *JAMA Internal Medicine* found that between 1999 and 2014, the percentage of Americans taking antidepressants has nearly doubled, from 6.8% to 12.7% of the population. Today, nearly 25 million adults in the U.S. have been taking antidepressants for at least two years.[30][31] Antidepressants, over time, may worsen anxiety and depression and can be more addictive than opioids.

Females are two and a half times as likely to take antidepressant medication as males. One in four women in their 40s and 50s are on drug treatment for depression.[32][33]

And, while there might be overuse of antidepressants in middle-aged women, young women who are menstruating but not sexually active are overprescribed birth control pills to treat conditions such as acne, cramps, heavy periods, headaches, and mood swings. Hormonal birth control (synthetic hormones) alleviates symptoms without treating the underlying problems. They can lead to mood disorders, depression, anxiety, and sleep disorders. It can be a vicious cycle.

When I was in my early to mid-forties, my periods became extremely heavy. Most premenopausal women go through this, and it is not fun. Heavy (and I mean heavy) periods are awful, and they are most definitely not convenient. I consulted with my OB-GYN, who told me that he could prescribe a birth control pill for me or an IUD to reduce menstrual bleeding. I will remind you that I was in my mid-forties. There was no need for me to go on any birth control as my husband had a vasectomy, and I really did not want the risks associated with synthetic hormones. The doctor insisted that birth control was the easiest and best option for me.

I got a second opinion, and the second OB-GYN that I saw started with recommending birth control pills as well. When I pressed on, she told me that endometrial ablation would be a good option without having to take any pills or do any hormones. Ablation is a procedure that involves destroying the uterine lining to reduce or stop menstrual flow altogether— basically, cauterizing the uterine lining. This is what I chose to have done. It was a very short procedure, in and out, with little to no pain and no medications. Period problem solved!

There are numerous risks and side effects associated with medications like antidepressants and birth control, but did you know that both also contribute to obesity? With nearly 71.6% of American adults ages 20 and older who are overweight and 40% being clinically obese, we do not need any more reasons as to why so many Americans are gaining weight.[34] Obesity is nothing to take lightly. Carrying all that extra weight around has some serious health consequences. It is linked to several health issues, including heart disease, diabetes, high blood pressure, and kidney disease. If current trends continue, estimates predict that by 2030, 50% of all men and women in the United States will be obese; not just overweight, but obese![35]

The body positivity movement has led us to believe that "big is beautiful." And this is not necessarily untrue. I believe there is beauty in all of us, big and small. But visceral fat is deadly. Can you really say that lethal fat—not just around your middle, but around your organs, which is linked to cancer, diabetes, and heart disease—is a thing of beauty? When being overweight and/or obese affects your health or, even worse, cuts your life short, the beauty in being big is questionable. It is hard to display body positivity when you can't bend down to tie your shoes or clip your toenails, do not have enough energy to climb a flight of stairs or play with your kids, are burdened with chronic illness, or even die an early death. I have known several individuals in their forties and fifties who, sadly, passed away from heart attacks due to severe obesity, leaving young children behind. These premature deaths that have cut lives short and leave loved ones behind are far from beautiful. Premature death, especially when it is preventable, is profoundly tragic.

Society is perhaps doing more harm than good when we no longer believe weight, BMI (body mass index), and body measurements should be ignored because they can hurt a person's feelings if the numbers appear unfavorable. All these numbers together tell a story, and even if they are unpleasant to hear, they should not be ignored.

The weight loss industry is a monster. Marketdata, LLC estimates that the total weight loss sales market in the United States is

GUIDANCE IN WELLNESS

around $90 BILLION and is still growing! 95% of diets fail, and yet we continue to fall for false promises because we all want a quick fix, a magic pill, or a potion. Do not be fooled by diet scammers selling the latest weight loss scheme and be very aware of chronic dieting. Suggesting that the best solution to weight loss and obesity is through pills or injections is a very dangerous approach. Not only are these so-called solutions typically very expensive, but they might help you lose a limited amount of weight only if you keep taking them. And the side effects can be costly.

During my first two years of college, I gained the notorious freshman fifteen. I hated those extra pounds, but between eating delivery pizza late at night with my roommate and working out a lot less than in my high school days, it was inevitable. I was eating more not-so-healthy foods and moving less. At the time, SlimFast was being advertised on television and seemed like a fantastic way for me to shed those unwanted pounds. The skinny and attractive women featured in TV commercials and magazines made SlimFast look like a miracle. The advertisements gave the impression that the "diet" was easy enough; one delicious shake for breakfast, one for lunch, and a "normal" dinner. After a few weeks of starving during the day and overeating at dinnertime, because I was famished, I was miserable and not making the progress I had hoped.

Since the SlimFast plan was giving me limited success in my weight loss journey, I decided to design and try my own plan which consisted of actual food within the same number of calories that the shakes offered. For breakfast, two scrambled eggs and a piece of toast with butter. For lunch, a half of a turkey or ham sandwich with mustard, tomato, lettuce, and onion, along with an apple. I was not starving by the time dinner rolled around, so my dinners were more in check with a sustainable calorie load. Watching portion sizes and being mindful of my eating habits worked, and the weight came off and has stayed off ever since.

I eat more today than I ever did in high school or college simply because of my love for CrossFit, daily walks with my dog, and active lifestyle with my family. Eating real food, getting enough macro- and micronutrients, and exercising have been sustainable habits for me to stick with for decades. This lifestyle has helped me keep my weight very consistent even through two pregnancies and the onset of menopause.

If the diet solutions promoted and advertised truly worked (not just for the short-term), everyone would be healthier and skinnier, but clearly, we are more overweight and obese than ever. We are doing something wrong. The pink drinks, the cleanses, the magic drops under the tongue, the protein powders and shakes that come in fruity pebble and s'mores flavors, the brightly colored energy teas, the pills and injections…they are all fooling you. If it sounds too good to be true, it is. Finding sustainable solutions in habits and lifestyle changes will offer better results and long-term success.

Even if you choose to eat real food and do not succumb to diet scammers, eating too little and restricting your diet too much is not good either. Women, in particular, who continuously follow severely low-calorie, "fad," or vegan diets often have the bone health of someone twice their age.

Studies have shown that 97% of dieters regain everything they have lost within three years.[36] Consult a certified nutritionist to help you determine what you should eat daily. You might need to eat more to successfully lose weight and maintain that weight loss. For example, I find that many of the women I work with are not getting enough protein or enough healthy fats in their diet. You need protein to maintain muscle, which promotes a healthy metabolism, and you need healthy fat to burn fat. If you deplete your body of what it needs, it will go into survival mode, slow your metabolism, and store fat.

Maintaining muscle mass while reducing body fat is important when you are on any diet, so be sure you are incorporating some sort of strength training into your routine along with sufficient protein to protect that valuable real estate.

Almost 17% of children in the United States are overweight, 20% are obese, and almost 6% are severely obese.[37] This is heartbreaking. When I was a kid going to school at Sentral of Fenton, there might have been a handful of kids (like 4 or 5) in the entire high school of 110 students who were overweight. Now, 4 out of 10 children are overweight or obese. No child should be faced with joint pain, respiratory issues, cardiovascular disease, and even the psychological effects that come with being overweight. Non-alcoholic fatty liver disease (too much fat in the liver cells) affects 10% of children in the general population and an estimated 36% of children with obesity and is on the rise. Children who are overweight or obese have an increased risk of obesity and related health problems as they enter adulthood. Childhood obesity is catastrophic and completely preventable.

A certain amount of body fat is essential because it provides energy, supports hormone production, and protects vital organs. But too much body fat can be deadly. There are two types of fat that help make up the human body. Visceral fat, which accumulates around the organs, poses several serious health risks, including cardiovascular disease, type 2 diabetes, fatty liver disease, and cancers. Subcutaneous fat is the fat we can see, which is located just under the skin. This is the fat that everyone wants to lose to look better in a swimsuit or a new outfit. Subcutaneous fat is the spare tire that most carry around their midsection.

Not only does a larger waist circumference affect how we look, but it can also be an indicator of excess visceral fat; the fat that surrounds our heart, liver, pancreas, and kidneys. A waist measurement over 40 inches (102 cm) in men and 35 inches (88 cm) in women suggests a higher amount of visceral fat. Waist size can be an effective measure for assessing obesity-related hypertension risk and is one of the most powerful ways to predict your risk for diabetes. If you want to find out if you are insulin resistant (pre-diabetic), simply take your waist measurement and divide it by your hip measurement. Measurements should be less than .8 for females or less than .9 for males.

Obesity most definitely contributes to high blood pressure along with excessive salt intake, lack of physical activity, and chronic stress. Approximately 116 million adults in the U.S., or nearly 47% of the adult population, have high blood pressure (hypertension).[38] High blood pressure is one of the most significant risk factors for heart disease, stroke, and kidney failure and is largely preventable through diet and lifestyle.

Statins prescribed to reduce cholesterol and indirectly manage high blood pressure are one of the most prescribed medications in the U.S., with millions of prescriptions written each year. It's estimated that around 30-45 million Americans are currently taking statins.

There is a strong link between the use of statins and developing type 2 diabetes. While statins are used to treat high cholesterol and high blood pressure, they are known to decrease insulin sensitivity, as well as insulin resistance—both significant factors for developing type 2 diabetes. Many patients find they need insulin after starting a statin, which is astonishing. Long-term statin use may unintentionally contribute to coronary artery calcification, potentially undermining its intended protective benefits. Niacin (B-3) is the most common and effective treatment that replaces statins. You can find natural sources of niacin in chicken, beef, pork and fatty fish, eggs, green leafy vegetables, and legumes. Talk to your doctor about ways to avoid statins.

Unlike type 1 diabetes, which is an autoimmune condition, type 2 diabetes is preventable. Type 2 diabetes is insulin resistance and is often linked to obesity, poor diet, and a sedentary lifestyle (or statin use). With the rise in obesity rates, type 2 diabetes has become a major public health issue. Type 2 diabetes is 100% preventable.

Elevated blood sugar also has a direct relationship to what is now being called type 3 diabetes: Alzheimer's. Alzheimer's is believed to result from a combination of genetic, environmental, and lifestyle factors. Cardiovascular health, poor sleep, chronic inflammation, and a neglected immune system play a part in this horrible neurodegenerative disorder, which affects over 6 million people in the country and over 50 million worldwide. If you could prevent this dreaded disease through diet and exercise, why wouldn't you?

We can also do our best to avoid cancer. Many cancers are preventable, as are type 2 diabetes and high blood pressure, with 48% of cancer cases attributed to obesity.[39] Obesity is linked to 13 types of cancer, including breast, colorectal, endometrial, liver, stomach, and thyroid. 20% of cancer cases are associated with chronic inflammation, 30% are linked to tobacco smoking and exposure to pollutants (such as asbestos), and 35% are related to dietary factors.[40][41] Again, there are a lot of cancers that are preventable, so why not do what you can to prevent such a fatal condition.

If you could avoid cancer from happening to you or your family, it is unquestionably worth a shot. So many people who get diagnosed with the dreaded "C word" regret not choosing a healthier lifestyle sooner. But no matter how hard you try, you cannot turn back time, so start now! Quit smoking, exercise, avoid ultra-processed foods, and consume healthy whole foods!

As a wellness coach certified in personal training and nutrition, it amazes me the advice that licensed physicians have given my clients or the information they are not told by their primary physician (like in the case of the woman on six prescription medications discussed earlier in this chapter). Here are some other real-life examples:

- A close friend of mine came to me for help after his doctor told him that he needed to lose weight. During our initial consultation, when I asked him what suggestions his doctor gave him to start his weight loss process, he told me that his doctor's recommendation was, "Try skipping breakfast. It works for me." Just because skipping breakfast works for the doctor does not mean it will work for his patient. What is the patient eating the rest of the day? How much are they eating at lunch and dinner? How many snacks are they eating and what are they? Are they exercising? Are they sleeping well? Are they constipated?

- A young male client communicated to me when I suggested that he quit drinking soda that his doctor assured him that "It was totally fine to drink one Mountain Dew every day. One soda a day was not going to hurt anything. Go ahead and enjoy your once-a-day pop." He was drinking a 20oz Mountain Dew daily, which has 73g of sugar (almost three times more than the daily allowance). The doctor did not ask what size of soda he was drinking every day. Even so, a regular 12oz Mountain Dew has 46g of sugar—still way too much for any person to consume in one day.

- A sixty-year-old woman sought out my help because she had suffered for decades from constipation and IBS. Doctors would suggest prescription laxatives, food plans, and nothing was working. She was a long-distance runner, ate a healthy diet, and was not overweight. But she was very bloated and very constipated; sometimes not pooping for weeks at a time.

Two weeks after meeting with me, after making some minor adjustments to her diet along with a few other suggestions, she was going to the bathroom regularly (without laxatives), lost two inches around her middle, and, as you can imagine, was feeling so much better.

- An existing client of mine referred a forty-year-old male friend of his to me. Turns out this new client's doctor was going to put him on a third medication to lower his triglycerides, which were sitting at 343. Triglycerides are a type of fat (lipid) found in your blood. When you eat, your body converts any calories it doesn't need to use right away into triglycerides. The triglycerides are stored in your fat cells. Later, hormones release triglycerides for energy between meals. The normal range for triglycerides is between 10 and 150. Unless this client got their numbers in line, more meds were in their future, and so their physician gave this client six months to get their triglycerides in check and requested a retest in six months before prescribing more medications. After making some adjustments to his diet and through some nutritional coaching, this client lowered his triglycerides to 115 within the six-month window their doctor gave them. Their doctor was amazed and asked them, "Who helped you reduce your overall numbers?" In fact, this person's numbers were so good across the board that their doctor took them off all prescription medications, and now they are prescription-free! Also, this client's doctor told him that his high blood pressure and cholesterol were hereditary and that he would need medication for the rest of his life. We proved that doctor wrong!

Generally, I spend one to two hours with every client during an initial consultation before creating their customized wellness plan because getting to know them is necessary to help them to the best of my ability. I ask a lot of questions, and I expect my clients to ask me a lot of questions, as they should. Their health is important, and they need to trust that I'm providing accurate advice and the correct information to help them reach their health goals.

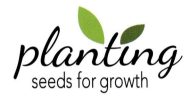

Your Primary Care Physician
Questions to Consider

1. What preventative care measures should I be taking?

2. Can you explain my diagnosis (if you have one) and what it means for my health?

3. Can I get bloodwork done as part of my annual physical (lipid test for cholesterol, triglycerides, and or a blood sugar test for glucose, etc.)?

4. What can I do to lower my blood pressure naturally?

5. What can I do to lower my triglycerides?

6. What can I do to lower my glucose levels?

7. How can I manage or improve my health with lifestyle changes?

8. When should I schedule my next appointment or follow-up?

9. What can I do to improve my overall health?

10. For any medications being prescribed:

- What is the purpose of this medication, and how does it work?

- How long do I need to be on this medication?

- What are some things I can do holistically to avoid taking this medication?

- Are there other options that have less risk or are safer?

- What are the known side effects, and what should I do if I experience them?

- Are there any specific instructions for taking this medication, such as timing, dietary restrictions, or interactions with other medications?

There are amazing doctors and brilliant scientists in the world and there are some incredible medications that are proven to be lifesaving. But, at the end of the day, you are the only person who can take care of you. Physical health is prevention, and it helps heal your body faster when you are faced with injury and illness. Good health is sustainable when you work at it, but you must be invested in your own journey to get there. No pill or procedure can do all the work for you.

Make sure you work with good doctors and caretakers. You owe it to yourself to be selective; hire a reputable primary physician. Be your own advocate. Always weigh the risks and the rewards when it comes to your options regarding medical care, especially when it comes to taking any prescription medication or undergoing any surgical procedure. And ask questions—a lot of them if you need to. You (or your insurance company) are paying for doctor visits, so get your money's worth. They get paid big bucks, so ask them important questions when you have their time and make sure you get answers. Write your questions down ahead of time and take them with you to your doctors' appointments to make sure you do not forget anything while you have your physician captive in the exam room. Your health is priceless, and you deserve more than a rushed five-minute appointment. You deserve personal care and the time needed when it comes to your life and the life of your loved ones.

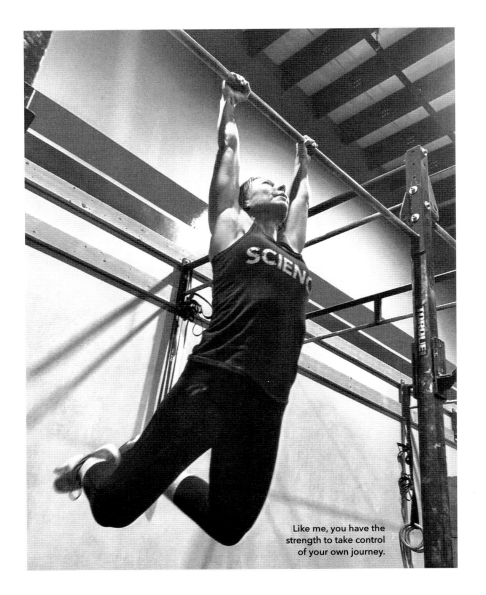

Like me, you have the strength to take control of your own journey.

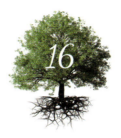

Lasting Impressions:
In the End

    In January 2018, Dad was complaining of severe low back and hip pain. After multiple chiropractor appointments and a few visits to his primary doctor, he was referred to a spine specialist who gave him a series of cortisone shots for what was diagnosed as bursitis of the hip.

    All of us girls and our families celebrated Easter with Mom and Dad back at the family acreage, and he still seemed to be struggling quite a bit with lower back and hip pain. I did not see Dad again until May of 2018 when he and Mom made a weekend trip to the Des Moines, Iowa area to visit me and my sister Sara. I knew immediately when I saw him get out of the car that he was suffering from something much worse than bursitis of the hip. He had dropped about ten pounds and could hardly walk; in fact, he almost fell a few times just trying to walk up our three front steps.

    Later that month, Dad decided to see a neurologist at the VA (United States Department of Veterans Affairs) and was diagnosed with non-Hodgkin lymphoma. PET scans and MRIs revealed a tumor in his lower back that had wrapped around his spine, causing the discomfort he had been having since the beginning of the year. His primary care doctor and spine specialist had been misdiagnosing Dad for months.

The VA said that because he served in Vietnam, his condition was likely caused by being exposed to Agent Orange. Agent Orange was a tactical herbicide used by the U.S. military during the Vietnam War. It was widely used to remove dense foliage and vegetation to expose enemy positions and clear areas for military operations. I remember Dad talking about his experiences in Vietnam and telling me how the jungles that he walked through with fellow U.S. Army soldiers were lush, thick, and green. But when aircraft would fly overhead to spray the chemical that blanketed the ground below, the jungles quickly turned brown and bare. He knew then that Agent Orange was some "potent shit," as he called it.

During the Vietnam War, the U.S. government believed that Agent Orange was safe for use in defoliation operations. However, subsequent research and evidence have shown that Agent Orange contained toxic chemicals, particularly dioxin, which have been linked to serious health effects in both military personnel and civilians exposed to it. Agent Orange was manufactured primarily by companies such as Dow Chemical and Monsanto under contract with the U.S. government during the Vietnam War. It just so happens that Monsanto produces Roundup® today, with the EPA reaffirming claims that there are "no risks of concern to human health from current uses of glyphosate" when it is used correctly.

After Dad's cancer diagnosis, he got a small check from the United States government that just screamed "guilt." Whether the "settlement" was a nice apology gift from the country that sent him to war (along with millions of others) and ultimately poisoned him or money to pay him off to keep him from suing the federal government, either way, the gesture had "guilty" written all over it.

Dad had surgery to remove the tumor and started cancer treatments immediately, both chemotherapy and radiation, and by the end of summer he was remarkably in remission and cancer-free. He started doing physical therapy daily to regain strength in his lower back and legs, which incurred substantial nerve damage from the delayed diagnosis. Along with the physical therapy and because Dad was healthy and in good shape before the cancer, eventually, Dad almost got back to his avid-gardening-and-deer-hunting-active self.

In fact, one year later, in October of 2019, Dad went back out into the Iowa wilderness to go deer hunting and successfully harvested himself a nice doe. Nothing spectacular like the huge white-tailed bucks that he was known for, but a deer nonetheless, and he was proud to have shot her, field-dressed her, dragged her out of the brush and got her home to butcher and eat. He was just so happy to be back to living his typical and active life.

During Thanksgiving that year (about one month after Dad shot that doe), Dad experienced the left side of his face falling and going numb. He and Mom were visiting my sister Sara and me in the Des Moines area for the holiday weekend, along with sisters Katie and Andrea and their families. He woke up on Saturday morning and his face definitely had a different appearance than the day before. Because it was a holiday weekend, Mom took him to a nearby walk-in clinic in Des Moines, where he was diagnosed with Bell's Palsy (acute facial palsy of unknown cause), given a steroid, and sent home. The doctor said that it might be two to three weeks before Dad's face would return to normal.

By mid-December, after waiting just over three weeks with no improvement—and even some worsening—of his facial condition, Dad made an appointment with the neurosurgeon who had performed his back surgery to remove that spinal tumor a year and a half earlier. His neurosurgeon prescribed a stronger dose of steroids for Bell's Palsy. Everyone hoped that the stronger dose would do the trick, and Dad would quickly be on the mend, as he and Mom had their first Caribbean cruise planned after the holidays.

Christmas had come and gone, and along with a drooping face, Dad started to experience severe pain. His face appeared worse than it was during the trip to his neurosurgeon a few weeks prior. So, the day before New Year's Eve, my sister Katie and Mom decided to take him to the emergency room at the Mayo Clinic in Rochester, Minnesota, to get some answers. Dad was admitted to the hospital that day so doctors could run some additional tests and investigate Dad's condition further. It was indeed a mystery. But, due to the holiday, we were told it could take a few days with medical personnel and physicians taking personal time off around the holidays.

Dad had been at Mayo for one day and on New Year's Eve, my husband and I drove up to the Mayo Clinic to be with Dad, who was in a hospital room. Mom and my sister Katie had stayed the night in a hotel directly across the street, which, of course, was unplanned due to the hecticness of the day before. New Year's Eve also happens to be my husband's and my wedding anniversary. Shortly after our arrival late that afternoon, a team of doctors (probably five or six of them) from the Mayo Clinic walked into Dad's hospital room to inform us that they were determined to find out what was wrong with Dad. Everyone on their team was committed to finding out what was causing his strange condition, which obviously was not Bell's Palsy.

On January 2, 2020, that same team of doctors who portrayed hope to us two days before came back for a visit and informed us that the cancer that plagued Dad in 2018 had returned. This time, the cancer appeared as tiny pin-sized lesions on the back of his brain, causing the left side of his face to droop, his left eyelid to remain open, and the onset of what would be rapid hearing loss in his left ear. The diagnosis was not good.

In March of 2020, Dad passed away. A few weeks before his passing, all of us girls and our families, including his nine grandchildren, gathered at the Brink family home on those three acres outside Fenton, Iowa, to have one last family barbecue, knowing that Dad was not going to live much longer. He had deteriorated to the point that not even a walker could get him from room to room anymore. The left side of his face had fallen severely; he had to wear a patch over his left eye to keep it from bulging and drying out. He had completely lost hearing out of his left ear and could hardly hear anything out of his right ear. His speech was even starting to slur so badly that we sometimes could not understand him. We had him use a whiteboard to write short messages for us when we had a tough time understanding what he wanted to say. And we used it to communicate with him since his hearing was all but gone. The cancer was not only restricting movements like walking and eating, but it was killing his nerves to all senses, and it was very evident.

At one point during the family gathering, I saw Dad sitting on the sofa finishing his meal and a glass of red wine. He loved a good barbecue and a nice cocktail: beer, wine, or a margarita. Dad truly appreciated good food and drink. When I walked into the living room, we made eye contact, and he motioned for me to come and sit next to him. I sat on his right side (his good side) close beside him. He put his hands on mine and said, "I've had such a good time with you, Amanda. I have enjoyed all these years with you and your sisters." I understood every word he said. They were as clear as day. No whiteboard needed. All I could do was look at him as tears swelled in my eyes as I squeezed his hand. "I love you, Dad," was all I could say. There was nothing more that needed to be said. The connection between father and daughter was raw and real.

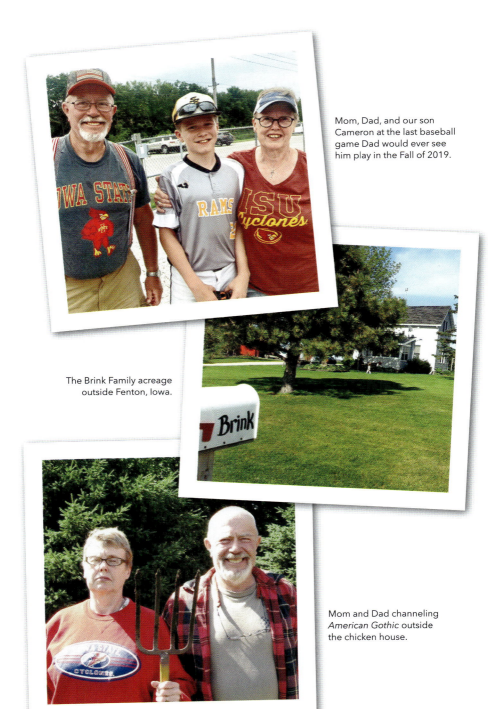

Mom, Dad, and our son Cameron at the last baseball game Dad would ever see him play in the Fall of 2019.

The Brink Family acreage outside Fenton, Iowa.

Mom and Dad channeling *American Gothic* outside the chicken house.

LASTING IMPRESSIONS   231

I look back on that moment with Dad and think about my roots there in that Iowa acreage where we shared so many great memories that I will cherish forever. Experiences and memories cultivated on hard work, homecooked meals, and time actively spent together as a family.

Knowing that I was so fortunate as a child in all the ways I've described in this book leads me to great sadness for so many families today that will never have what the Brink girls had. We might not have had a lot of money growing up, but we were rich in countless other ways. So many families today rely on convenience and short-cuts. Kids depend on handouts from their parents and are overcoddled and disconnected from one another by an even stronger connection to personal digital devices and video games. Most families are overfed yet malnourished, eating a diet of prepackaged processed food stripped of organic nutrients and created in a factory, and not getting the nutrition they need from home-cooked meals. Gathering for family mealtime is a thing of the past. We are pushed a prescription for every symptom known to man versus fixing our health problems and tackling the root of the cause (which, in most cases, is nutrition and fitness-based).

With modern technology and advancements, we have forgotten the basics. I challenge each and every one of you to return to the basics—the roots of what truly worked. There is no research paper or science experiment that can tell us what we already know. Active living, moving more, eating real food, reducing stress, getting enough sleep, challenging yourself, and connecting with family and good friends—that is what builds a long, healthy life.

When you get to the point in your life where you are looking back on all the years you have lived (and all of us will get there at some point), will you have any regrets? Or will you be satisfied with how you spent your moments here on this earth?

Will you wish you had spent more hours at the office, scrolling through social media, or watching the news? Or will you be grateful for all the time you spent with those you love and doing good things? Will you wish you had quit smoking sooner or eaten better? Or will you be thankful for a healthy life that you were able to enjoy to the fullest?

We all get one shot. We all have one body that should be treated like a gift from God because it is. Each one of us has only one life to live. Life is not a dress rehearsal.

Even though Dad died of cancer, he got life right.

In true CrossFit fashion, I created a Hero WOD for Dad. A Hero WOD (Workout of the Day) is an intense and challenging workout that is supposed to remind us of the hardships and sacrifices made by military members or first responders. I, along with roughly fifty or so fellow CrossFitters from across the country, got outside and did a workout to celebrate Dad on his birthday that year, which just so happens to be Earth Day (very fitting for a man who loved the outdoors). It was surreal, and I appreciate every single one of those who joined me that morning of April 22, 2020. Feel free to honor my dad by accomplishing the workout below. I do it every year on his birthday.

Barn Dog 2020: a Hero WOD for a Vietnam Vet and a Wonderful Father

Dad's birthday was April 22, which is Earth Day. Pretty fitting for a guy who loved planting gardens and trees and taking care of God's creatures. In honor of his life and in true CrossFit fashion, I put together a Hero WOD in his name the year he passed away.

"Barn Dog" is a Hero WOD in honor of Thomas (Barney) Brink

(4/22/47 – 3/23/20), a US Army Veteran. For time (in order) with a weighted vest 14/20lbs.

- 91 Walking Lunges
- 47 Over-the-Shoulder Sandbag Throws (40/60lbs)
- 91 Walking Lunges
- 67 Kettlebell Swings (35/53lbs)
- 91 Walking Lunges
- 73 Hand Release Push-ups
- 91 Walking Lunges

The four rounds of walking lunges represent the birth month Barney was born and the four strong women he helped raise. The 364 total walking lunges represent the number of days Barney fought in the Vietnam War. The 47 over-the-shoulder sandbag throws represent his birth year and the number of years he was married to his faithful wife, Susan (anniversary 2/16/73). 67 was the year Barney was honorably discharged from the US Army from active duty. And 73 represents the year Barney married Susan and what would have been his 73rd birthday on 4/22/20 (Earth Day).

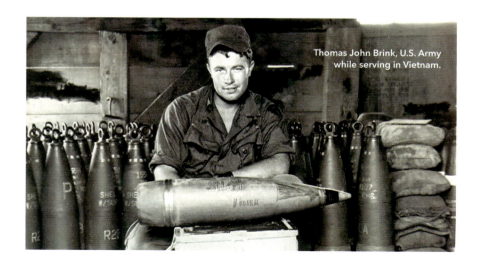

Thomas John Brink, U.S. Army while serving in Vietnam.

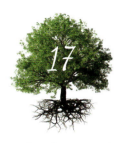

Final Thoughts:
Walking the Walk and Living Wellness

My entire life (from birth to the present) has been based on the notion that the body is completely capable of building natural immunity. My parents believed in gardening, hunting, and raising poultry and pigs for consumption. I even remember, as a very small child, my mother milking goats by hand so we would have vitamin-rich milk to pour over breakfast cereal in the mornings. Mom and Dad believed in enjoying the outdoors often and getting dirty by hard work and play.

My parents had three acres where my dad cultivated two gigantic gardens that produced enough vegetables for at least a year with enough leftovers to share with friends and family. We would eat fresh vegetables in season and then freeze and can what we could not eat during the harvest months. My dad also had apple and pear trees, raspberry bushes, and strawberry plants for fresh fruit and for homemade jams and jellies that my mom would make and store in our pantry for all-year-round enjoyment. Current, crabapple and

FINAL THOUGHTS

235

raspberry jams made the best topping on her home-baked bread.

My dad also taught all four of his daughters to hunt pheasants and deer. We would always consume what was killed, never wasting an ounce. Our family of six enjoyed deer roasts that Dad would carefully season and slow cook on Sundays for a big after-church meal. Deer sticks and jerky were a crowd favorite at gatherings and for easy snacks while we girls were in sports. Pheasant breasts and the occasional wood duck were also delicious menu options. Dad loved bow hunting turkey in the spring, which always provided a challenging pursuit, and in the end, the large birds would make several servings of nutritious turkey for us all to enjoy.

Dad also raised his own pigs for slaughter and twenty or more broiler chickens every summer for butchering. This was because he worked at a grain elevator for most of his life, where he was introduced to the chemicals and pharmaceutical drugs that farmers mixed into feed and fed to confinement livestock. Dad believed that the drugs commonly mixed with animal feed were dangerous and should not be consumed by people, even indirectly through the meats we eat.

My parents took great care in raising their four daughters. Great care in providing for us the best way they knew how with what they had. We were brought up to work hard, care for the Earth and the creatures on it, and appreciate what God has given us.

My children have been taught from a very early age how to prepare nutritious meals that are well-balanced and have all the nutrients they need to grow healthy and strong and maintain optimum health as young adults. Ingredients are the first thing we read on nutrition labels, and if we cannot pronounce any of them, we do not consume them. I food prep every weekend to be sure we are well-prepared for the coming week between work and school schedules, sporting events, and daily workouts. And every night, our family enjoys a thoughtful, home-prepared meal around the table.

I have a sincere belief that stems from my childhood that the body (if given enough natural and organic nutrients) can heal itself without any artificial or genetically modified materials. This includes everything from preservatives to most medications and vaccines.

I do not take supplements, and rarely do I ever take even Tylenol. In fact, I have never even taken painkillers prescribed to me by doctors for the following: two C-sections, surgery to take out a tumor on my right ovary, hand surgery for a broken finger that included three pins, a bone spur that was chiseled off my forehead, and vaginal ablation. I have a strong belief that inflammation in the body is controlled by what we consume daily. Artificial ingredients and chemicals found in processed foods, along with refined sugars and bleached flours, all play a role in how inflammation affects our bodies.

People who know me know that health is a top priority, not only in my life, but that I strongly encourage others to strive to be their healthiest. I am always willing to help others find healthier ways to prevent sickness and inflammation. Organic and holistic is my life. I talk the talk, and I walk the walk. Just ask anyone who knows me.

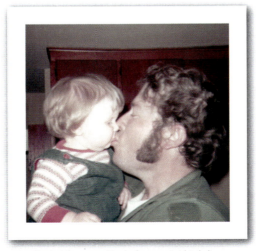

Dad giving me a kiss before my 1st birthday.

The Why Behind the How

I wrote this book to empower people with the knowledge and tools to take control of their health, cutting through the noise of misleading marketing that promises quick fixes. My goal is to help motivate and inspire others to lay a foundation for sustainable well-being. While I'm not a doctor or scientist, I've lived a life focused on health and wellness, and I know firsthand the power of feeling your best and living a productive, successful life.

With certifications in nutrition, personal training, and health coaching and a master's degree in industrial and organizational psychology, I have the expertise to guide others on their wellness journey. I've served on boards from Iowa to Washington, DC and spoken at national conferences alongside experts like Dr. Mehmet Oz. My commitment to wellness earned me a nomination as a Hearst Wellness Champion from 2018 to 2021 in addition to my role as General Sales Manager at the Hearst CBS affiliate in Des Moines, Iowa. Today, I continue my passion for health by volunteering as a wellness advocate on the WellWorks! Committee at Strategic America and coaching individuals on their nutrition and fitness.

In 2020, I founded Hull Health, initially sharing wellness tips, workout ideas, and healthy recipes on social media during the pandemic. Since then, my mission has expanded to address the health needs of individuals, organizations, and communities. For more information, you can find me on social media or visit my website at hull-health.com.

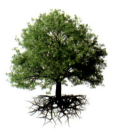

Notes

1. Precedence Research. "U.S. Protein Supplements Market Size to Surpass USD 9.69 Billion in 2023 and Estimated to Reach USD 21.97 Billion by 2033." Precedence Research, https://www.precedenceresearch.com/us-protein-supplements-market.

2. Harvard Medical School. "Sugar and the Brain." Harvard Medical School, https://hms.harvard.edu/news-events/publications-archive/brain/sugar-brain.

3. American Heart Association. "How Much Sugar Is Too Much?" https://www.heart.org/en/healthy-living/healthy-eating/eat-smart/sugar/how-much-sugar-is-too-much.

4. Tittgemeyer, M., et al. "Food Addiction: The Link Between Ultra-Processed Foods and Addictive Behaviors." *British Medical Journal*, 2023.

5. "How Volunteering Improves Health and Well-being," Harvard Health Blog, https://www.health.harvard.edu.

6. "15 Reasons Why People With Depression Don't Get Treatment," *Psychology Today*. Retrieved from https://www.psychologytoday.com.

NOTES

7. Lisa Marshall and Nicholas Goda, "Melatonin Use Soars Among Children, with Unknown Risks," *CU Boulder Today*, November 13, 2023, https://www.colorado.edu/today/2023/11/13/melatonin-use-soars-among-children-unknown-risks.

8. "More than 4 in 10 U.S. Workers Don't Take All Their Paid Time Off," Pew Research Center, August 10, 2023, https://www.pewresearch.org/short-reads/2023/08/10/more-than-4-in-10-u-s-workers-dont-take-all-their-paid-time-off.

9. "2023 Survey Reveals American Dining Out Habits," U.S. Foods, https://www.usfoods.com/our-services/business-trends/american-dining-out-habits-2023.html.

10. Cleveland Clinic, "Can too Much Tech Cause ADHD in Your Child?" health.clevelandclinic.org.

11. Cleveland Clinic, "ADHD and Kids" Podcast episode, Health Essentials Podcast.

12. American Psychological Association, "The Impact of Checking Social Media on Mental Health," APA.org.

13. Psychology Today, "How Smartphone Addiction Affects Mental Health," *Psychology Today*.

14. "Snack Food Industry Accounts for 27% of All Food & Beverage Sales," SNAC International, 2023, https://candyusa.com/cst/snack-food-industry-accounts-for-27-of-all-food-beverage-sales.

15. "Ultra-Processed Foods Account for More than Half of Calories Consumed at Home," Johns Hopkins Bloomberg School of Public Health, November 2023, https://publichealth.jhu.edu/2024/ultraprocessed-foods-account-for-more-than-half-of-calories-consumed-at-home.

16. "Ultra-Processed Diet Leads to Extra Calories, Weight Gain," NIH Director's Blog, May 21, 2019, https://directorsblog.nih.gov/2019/05/21/ultra-processed-diet-leads-to-extra-calories-weight-gain.

17. "Energy & Sports Drinks - Global," Statista Market Forecast, https://www.statista.com/outlook/cmo/non-alcoholic-drinks/soft-drinks/energy-sports-drinks/worldwide; "Energy & Sports Drinks - US," Statista Market Forecast, https://www.statista.com/outlook/cmo/non-alcoholic-drinks/soft-drinks/energy-sports-drinks/united-states.

18. "Use of PFAS in Cosmetics 'Widespread,' New Study Finds," University of Notre Dame, https://news.nd.edu/news/use-of-pfas-in-cosmetics-widespread-new-study-finds.

19. "Phthalates," Breast Cancer Prevention Partners, https://www.bcpp.org/resource/phthalates.

20. Adams, Kelly M., W. Scott Butsch, and Martin Kohlmeier. "The State of Nutrition Education at US Medical Schools." *Journal of Biomedical Education*, vol. 2015, Article ID 452826, 2015. https://doi.org/10.1155/2015/452826.

21. Centers for Medicare & Medicaid Services (CMS), "National Health Expenditure Fact Sheet," CMS, last modified December 18, 2024, https://www.cms.gov/data-research/statistics-trends-and-reports/national-health-expenditure-data/nhe-fact-sheet.

22. "U.S. Healthcare Spending Rose 7.5% in 2023, Government Report Says," Reuters, December 18, 2024, https://www.reuters.com/business/healthcare-pharmaceuticals/us-healthcare-spending-rose-75-2023-government-report-says-2024-12-18.

23. Centers for Disease Control and Prevention (CDC), "Unnecessary Antibiotic Prescribing in U.S. Ambulatory Care Settings," *Journal of the American Medical Association*, 315, no. 17 (2016): 1864–1873, https://jamanetwork.com/journals/jama/fullarticle/2518263.

24. Centers for Disease Control and Prevention (CDC), "Antibiotic Resistance Threats in the United States, 2019," CDC, last modified November 13, 2019, https://www.cdc.gov/antimicrobial-resistance/data-research/threats/index.html.

25. National Institute of Diabetes and Digestive and Kidney Diseases (NIDDK), "Digestive Diseases Statistics for the United States," NIDDK, last modified December 2024, https://www.niddk.nih.gov/health-information/health-statistics/digestive-diseases.

26. National Institute of Diabetes and Digestive and Kidney Diseases (NIDDK). "Heartburn."

27. Endo-World. "Gastroesophageal Reflux Disease, Hiatal Hernia, and Heartburn."

NOTES

28. Centers for Disease Control and Prevention (CDC), "Antidepressant Use Among Adults: United States, 2015–2018," National Center for Health Statistics Data Brief No. 377 (2020), https://www.cdc.gov/nchs/products/databriefs/db377.htm.

29. National Women's Health Network, "Older Women Use the Most Antidepressants, Survey Finds," National Women's Health Network, last modified December 2022, https://www.npwomenshealthcare.com/older-women-use-the-most-antidepressants-survey-finds.

30. National Center for Health Statistics (NCHS). "Antidepressant Use Among U.S. Adults."

31. Behavioral Health News. "Antidepressants: A Complicated Picture."

32. National Center for Health Statistics (NCHS). "Trends in Antidepressant Use in the United States." Centers for Disease Control and Prevention.

33. NIMH (National Institute of Mental Health). "Mental Health Medications."

34. Linda Searing, "About 74 Percent of Adults in the U.S. Are Overweight, According to the CDC," *The Washington Post*, last modified December 2023, https://www.washingtonpost.com/health/2023/12/15/overweight-adults-cdc.

35. Melissa Healy, "By 2030, Nearly Half of U.S. Adults Will Be Obese, Experts Predict," *Los Angeles Times*, last modified December 18, 2019, https://www.latimes.com/science/story/2019-12-18/obesity-rate-projections-2030.

36. "Statistics," Center of Excellence for Eating Disorders, University of North Carolina at Chapel Hill, accessed December 26, 2024, https://www.med.unc.edu/psych/eatingdisorders/learn-more/about-eating-disorders/statistics.

37. Centers for Disease Control and Prevention (CDC), "Health E-Stats: Prevalence of Overweight, Obesity, and Severe Obesity Among Children and Adolescents Aged 2–19 Years: United States, 2017–2018," National Center for Health Statistics, last modified December 2020, https://www.cdc.gov/nchs/data/hestat/obesity-child-17-18/obesity-child.htm.

38. Centers for Disease Control and Prevention (CDC), "High Blood Pressure Facts," CDC, last modified May 15, 2024, https://www.cdc.gov/high-blood-pressure/data-research/facts-stats/index.html.

39. National Cancer Institute, "Obesity and Cancer Fact Sheet," National Cancer Institute, last modified December 2023, https://www.cancer.gov/about-cancer/causes-prevention/risk/obesity/obesity-fact-sheet.

40. "Obesity and Cancer," Centers for Disease Control and Prevention, last modified January 2023, https://www.cdc.gov/cancer/risk-factors/obesity.html.

41. "Cancer Risk Factors," American Cancer Society, last modified September 2023, https://www.cancer.org/cancer/risk-prevention.html.